simply
smoothies

Fresh & Fast Diabetes-Friendly
Snacks & Complete Meals

LINDA GASS

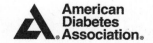

American
Diabetes
Association®

Director, Book Publishing, Abe Ogden; *Managing Editor,* Greg Guthrie; *Acquisitions Editor,* Victor Van Beuren; *Production Manager,* Melissa Sprott; *Composition,* ADA; *Production Services,* Cenveo Publisher Services, Inc.; *Cover Design,* Jody Billert; *Printer,* Versa Press.

Printed in the United States of America
1 3 5 7 9 10 8 6 4 2

The suggestions and information contained in this publication are generally consistent with the *Clinical Practice Recommendations* and other policies of the American Diabetes Association, but they do not represent the policy or position of the Association or any of its boards or committees. Reasonable steps have been taken to ensure the accuracy of the information presented. However, the American Diabetes Association cannot ensure the safety or efficacy of any product or service described in this publication. Individuals are advised to consult a physician or other appropriate health care professional before undertaking any diet or exercise program or taking any medication referred to in this publication. Professionals must use and apply their own professional judgment, experience, and training and should not rely solely on the information contained in this publication before prescribing any diet, exercise, or medication. The American Diabetes Association— its officers, directors, employees, volunteers, and members—assumes no responsibility or liability for personal or other injury, loss, or damage that may result from the suggestions or information in this publication.

∞ The paper in this publication meets the requirements of the ANSI Standard Z39.48-1992 (permanence of paper).

ADA titles may be purchased for business or promotional use or for special sales. To purchase more than 50 copies of this book at a discount, or for custom editions of this book with your logo, contact the American Diabetes Association at the address below, at booksales@diabetes.org, or by calling 703-299-2046.

American Diabetes Association
1701 North Beauregard Street
Alexandria, Virginia 22311

DOI: 10.2337/9781580405270

Library of Congress Cataloging-in-Publication Data
Gassenheimer, Linda.
 Simply smoothies / Linda Gassenheimer.
     pages cm
 Includes bibliographical references and index.
 ISBN 978-1-58040-527-0 (alkaline paper) 1. Smoothies (Beverages) 2. Quick and easy cooking. 3. Diabetes–Diet therapy–Recipes. 4. Blenders (Cooking) I. American Diabetes Association. II. Title.
  TX815.G37 2014
  641.5'55--dc23
                         2013031872

To my husband, Harold,
for his love,
constant enthusiasm for my work,
and support.

Contents

Acknowledgments

One of the best parts of writing a book is working with so many talented and friendly people. I'd like to thank them all for their enthusiastic support.

My biggest thank you goes to my husband, Harold, who encouraged me, helped me test every recipe, and spent hours helping me edit every word. His constant encouragement for all of my work has made this book a partnership.

Thank you to Abe Ogden, director of book publishing at the American Diabetes Association, for his guidance and support. He worked closely with me to enable this book to come to life.

I'd also like to thank Greg Guthrie, Managing Editor at the American Diabetes Association, for his wonderful work in managing this book. Thanks also to Melissa Sprott, Production Manager, for creating the beautiful design for this book.

Thank you to my Miami Herald editor, Kathy Martin, for her constant support of my "Dinner in Minutes" column.

Thank you to Joseph Cooper and Bonnie Berman, hosts of "Topical Currents," and to the staff at WLRN National Public Radio for their help and enthusiasm for my weekly "Food News and Views" segment.

I'd also like to thank my family, who have supported my projects and encouraged me every step of the way: my son James, his wife Patty, and their children Zachary, Jacob, and Haley; my son John, his wife Jill, and their children Jeffrey and Joanna; my son Charles, his wife Lori, and their sons Daniel and Matthew; and my sister Roberta and her husband Robert.

And, finally, thank you to all of my readers and listeners who have written and called over the years. You have helped shape my ideas and made the solitary task of writing a two-way street.

Introduction: Simply Smoothies—In Minutes!

Refreshing Breakfasts, Lunches, and Snacks Blended to Perfection

Looking for a quick breakfast, lunch, or snack? Something you can whip up in minutes and maybe take on the go? You'll find 60 smoothie choices here with a variety of flavors and textures to please your every mood. They're all quick and easy.

For breakfast on the run, a quick lunch, or a simple snack, you can assemble the ingredients in a blender jar and store it in the refrigerator. All you need to do is power up the blender and take your complete meal or snack with you.

There's a lot of variety. Choose from fruit-based smoothies like the Blackberry Breeze, Peanut Butter Banana, or Pear Cinnamon for breakfast. Savor a Cantaloupe Crush, Curried Gazpacho, or Pear Avocado Passion for lunch. If you're looking for a quick snack during the day, Double Chocolate Raspberry Treat, Apple Pie Perfect, or Espresso Crema might fill the bill.

Shopping

Many of these smoothies are made with frozen, unsweetened fruits. You can keep these fruits on hand to assemble these smoothies quickly. Consider keeping other ingredients on hand as well to help you make great meals in minutes. For example, almonds, walnuts, pecans, and other nuts are a good source of protein and are used in several recipes in this book. You can keep nuts in the freezer to use when needed.

Pasteurized, liquid egg whites can be found in cartons in the supermarket. They add a good source of protein to many of these smoothies without altering the flavor profile of the smoothie.

Flax seeds contain omega-3 fatty acids and have high levels of dietary fiber. Several brands are gluten free. If you are looking for a gluten-free product, read the labels to be sure. Whey protein powder is another source of protein added to some of the smoothies in this book.

All of the smoothie recipes in this book require few ingredients, and the shopping is easy, too. All of the ingredients can be found in a local supermarket.

Breakfast

Wake up your morning taste buds with enticing breakfast smoothies. Maybe it's a coffee or mocha flavor you're in the mood for. Try the Cappuccino Smoothie made with instant espresso or the Mocha Magic Smoothie made with frozen chocolate yogurt. Peanut butter and bananas are my childhood favorite. They both come together in a Peanut Butter Banana Smoothie. The fruit based smoothies, like Cherry Berry Smoothie and Nutty Peach Whip, are colorful and sweet. Or, you can wake up your morning taste buds with the spicy Virgin Bloody Mary Smoothie.

Lunch

Savory and sweet, these lunch smoothies make a delicious, filling lunch. Each one is a complete meal. Enjoy a hint of India with the Mango Lassi Smoothie or Curried Gazpacho Smoothie. Looking for a peanut-butter-and-jelly fix? The Nutty Butter Blizzard Smoothie is your answer. For Italian flavors, try the Pesto Pizzazz Smoothie, usher in autumn with the Pumpkin Pleaser Smoothie, or tingle your taste buds with the Red Pepper Popper Smoothie.

Snacks

Getting hungry before lunch around 11:00 a.m. or in the afternoon around 4:00 p.m.? Try some snacks to savor. Apple Pie Perfect Smoothie, Key Lime Smoothie, or Chai Spice 'n' Nice Smoothie will give you a lift.

Equipment

There are many brands of blenders and many have different strengths and speeds. To make sure your smoothie has the right texture, I have included both timing and texture notes. Follow both for the best results. The smoothies should be smooth. This may take a few more or a few less seconds in your blender.

Shop Smart

To help assemble these smoothies in minutes, I have designed these recipes using ingredients you can find at your supermarket. This guide isn't a specific recommendation of any particular brand. You can choose from the many options available. The key is to *shop smart* by looking at the nutrition information provided in this section. I have listed the items for which I have found a range of products with variations in calorie, fat, carbohydrate, or sodium content to guide you toward healthy options. You may not find the exact values. Use this information as a guideline for what you choose.

Many of these items can be kept on hand so that you only have to shop for a few fresh ingredients.

Look for the following:

- Unsweetened almond milk with 3.0 g fat, 2.0 g carbohydrates per cup

- Biscotti with 100 calories, 5.0 g fat, 15.0 g carbohydrates, 75 mg sodium (such as Starbucks Vanilla Almond Biscotti)

- Carrot juice with 94 calories, 21.9 g carbohydrates, 156 mg sodium per cup

- Cracker meal with 440 calories, 2.0 g fat, 10.7 g protein, 93.0 g carbohydrates, 18.0 g sodium per cup

- Swiss cheese (such as light Laughing Cow Wedges) with 35 calories, 2.0 g fat, 2.5 g protein, 260 mg sodium for 3/4-ounce piece

- Desiccated coconut flakes (sweetened) with 388 calories, 24.0 g fat, 44.1 g carbohydrates, 242 mg sodium per cup

- Diet soda with 0 calories, 0–80 mg sodium per cup

- Flaxseed meal with 37 calories, 2.9 g fat, 1.3 g protein, 2.0 g carbohydrates per tablespoon

- Low-sugar grape jam with 56 calories, 13.8 g carbohydrates per tablespoon

- Spreadable fruit with 30 calories, 8.0 g carbohydrates per tablespoon

- Lemonade frozen concentrate with 72 calories, 18.2 g carbohydrates per fluid ounce

- Light coconut milk with 135 calories, 13.3 g fat, 3.0 g protein, 9.0 g carbohydrates, 60 mg sodium per cup

- Nonfat yogurt with 103 calories, 4.0 g fat, 9.3 g protein, 18.1 g carbohydrates, 142 mg sodium per cup

- Low-fat yogurt with 154 calories, 3.8 g fat, 12.9 g protein, 17.3 g carbohydrates, 172 mg sodium per cup

- Low-fat vanilla or fruit-flavored yogurt (not fruit on the bottom) with 208 calories, 3.1 g fat, 12.1 g protein, 33.8 g carbohydrates, 162 mg sodium per cup

- Nonfat vanilla or fruit-flavored yogurt with 140 calories, 16.0 g protein, 17.0 g carbohydrates, 75 mg sodium per 6-ounce carton

- Low-fat no-salt-added cottage cheese with 163 calories, 2.3 g fat, 28.0 g protein, 6.1 g carbohydrates, 29 mg sodium per cup

- Low-sodium tomato juice with 41 calories, 10.3 g carbohydrates, 24 mg sodium per cup

- Nonfat ricotta cheese with 200 calories, 20.0 g protein, 20.0 g carbohydrates, 260 mg sodium per cup

- Canned passion fruit nectar with 18.8 calories, 4.8 g carbohydrates per fluid ounce

- Pasteurized, liquid egg whites with 6 calories, 1.0 g fat, 1.0 g protein, 11 mg sodium per tablespoon

- Nonfat sour cream with 9 calories, 0.4 g protein, 1.9 g carbohydrates, 17 mg sodium per tablespoon

- Reduced-fat sour cream with 18 calories, 1.0 g fat, 1.0 g protein, 1.0 g carbohydrates, 13 mg sodium per tablespoon

- Soft tofu with 151 calories, 9.2 g fat, 16.2 g protein, 4.5 g carbohydrates, 20 mg sodium per cup

- Sugar substitute of your choice (I have used several different brands in creating the recipes.)

- Sunbutter with 100 calories, 8.0 g fat, 3.5 g protein, 3.5 carbohydrates, 60 mg sodium per tablespoon

- Toasted wheat germ with 27 calories, 0.8 g fat, 2.0 g protein, 3.5 g carbohydrates, 0 mg sodium per tablespoon

- Light chocolate-flavored soymilk with 90 calories, 1.5 g fat, 3.0 g protein, 16.0 g carbohydrates (14 g sugar), 85 mg sodium per cup (such as Silk)

- Light vanilla soymilk with 70 calories, 1.5 g fat, 6.0 g protein, 7.0 g carbohydrates (5 g sugar), 110 mg sodium per cup (such as Silk)

- Vanilla whey protein powder with 80 calories, 1.1 g fat, 16.0 g protein, 1.0 g carbohydrates, 65 mg sodium per 3/4 ounce

Breakfast

Banana Grape Smoothie

*The banana and grapes sweeten this quick smoothie. It can
be made a day ahead and stored in the refrigerator.*

Helpful Hints

- Ground flaxseed can be used instead of flaxseed meal.
- Store flaxseed in the refrigerator to keep it from becoming rancid.

1/2 cup ripe banana, sliced
1/2 cup seedless red or black grapes
1 cup light vanilla soymilk (such as Silk)
2 tablespoons flaxseed meal
1 scoop (3/4 ounce) vanilla whey protein powder

- Place banana, grapes, soymilk, flaxseed, and whey protein powder in a blender.

- Blend on high for 30 seconds or until smooth.

Makes one 16-ounce smoothie.

Exchanges/Food Choices: 2 fruit, 1 carbohydrate, 2 lean protein, 2 fat
Per serving: Calories 350, Calories from Fat 90, Total Fat 10 g, Saturated Fat 1.5 g,
Trans Fat 0 g, Cholesterol 50 mg, Sodium 190 mg, Potassium 880 mg,
Total Carbohydrate 42 g, Dietary Fiber 8 g, Sugars 21 g, Protein 26 g, Phosphorus 368 mg

Shopping List:

1 ripe banana
1 small bunch seedless red or black
  grapes
1 carton light vanilla soymilk

Staples:

flaxseed meal
vanilla whey protein powder

Shop Smart

- Light vanilla soymilk with 70 calories, 1.5 g fat, 6.0 g protein, 7.0 g carbohydrates (5 g sugar), 110 mg sodium per cup (such as Silk)
- Flaxseed meal with 37 calories, 2.9 g fat, 1.3 g protein, 2.0 g carbohydrates per tablespoon
- Vanilla whey protein powder with 80 calories, 1.1 g fat, 16.0 g protein, 1.0 g carbohydrates, 65 mg sodium per 3/4 ounce

Apple Blackberry Smoothie

*Memories of picking wild blackberries and enjoying crisp apples
in autumn prompted me to create this smoothie.*

Helpful Hints

- Ground flaxseed can be used instead of flaxseed meal.
- Use frozen blackberries not packed in sugar syrup.
- Pasteurized, liquid egg whites can be found in cartons in the dairy/egg case.
- Store flaxseed in the refrigerator to keep it from becoming rancid.

1/2 cup apple with skin, cubed
1/2 cup frozen, unsweetened blackberries
1 tablespoon flaxseed meal
3/4 cup low-fat vanilla yogurt
1 teaspoon ground cinnamon
1/2 cup pasteurized, liquid egg whites
1 tablespoon unsalted walnuts

- Cut apple into small pieces.

- Place apple in a blender with the blackberries, flaxseed meal, yogurt, cinnamon, egg whites, and walnuts.

- Blend on high 45 seconds or until smooth.

Makes one 12-ounce smoothie.

*Exchanges/Food Choices: 3 fruit, 1 fat-free milk, 2 lean protein, 2 fat
Per serving: Calories 470, Calories from Fat 140, Total Fat 15 g, Saturated Fat 2 g,
Trans Fat 0 g, Cholesterol 10 mg, Sodium 320 mg, Potassium 640 mg,
Total Carbohydrate 59 g, Dietary Fiber 11 g, Sugars 46 g, Protein 27 g, Phosphorus 285 mg*

Shopping List:

1 apple
1 package frozen, unsweetened
   blackberries
1 carton low-fat vanilla yogurt
1 package unsalted walnuts

Staples:

flaxseed meal
ground cinnamon
pasteurized, liquid egg whites

Shop Smart

- Flaxseed meal with 37.0 calories, 2.9 g fat, 1.3 g protein, 2.0 g carbohydrates per tablespoon
- Low-fat vanilla or fruit-flavored yogurt (not fruit on the bottom) with 208 calories, 3.1 g fat, 12.1 g protein, 33.8 g carbohydrates, 162 mg sodium per cup
- Pasteurized, liquid egg whites with 6 calories, 1.0 g fat, 1.0 g protein, 11 mg sodium per tablespoon

Banana Strawberry Smoothie

When my bananas are very ripe, I like to freeze a few. They're perfect for this smoothie, giving flavor along with the strawberries to this tofu- and soymilk-based smoothie.

This smoothie can be made the night before and refrigerated until needed. Stir once before serving.

Helpful Hints

- Fresh ripe bananas can be used instead of frozen.
- Firm tofu can be used instead of soft.
- Use frozen strawberries that are not in sugar syrup.

1/4 cup plain soft tofu
1/2 cup frozen, ripe banana slices
1/4 cup frozen, unsweetened strawberries
1 cup light vanilla soymilk (such as Silk)
1 teaspoon vanilla extract
1 scoop (3/4 ounce) vanilla whey protein powder
Sugar substitute equivalent to 2 teaspoons sugar (optional)

- Place tofu, banana slices, strawberries, soymilk, vanilla extract, whey protein powder, and sugar substitute (optional) in a blender.

- Blend 1 minute or until smooth.

Makes one 18-ounce smoothie.

Exchanges/Food Choices: 3 carbohydrate, 3 lean protein, 1 fat
Per serving: Calories 370, Calories from Fat 110, Total Fat 12 g, Saturated Fat 2 g,
Trans Fat 0 g, Cholesterol 50 mg, Sodium 200 mg, Potassium 920 mg,
Total Carbohydrate 37 g, Dietary Fiber 8 g, Sugars 14 g, Protein 30 g, Phosphorus 415 mg

Shopping List:

1 package plain soft tofu
1 ripe banana
1 package frozen, unsweetened
   strawberries
1 carton light vanilla soymilk

Staples:

vanilla whey protein powder
sugar substitute

Shop Smart

- Soft tofu with 151 calories, 9.2 g fat, 16.2 g protein, 4.5 g carbohydrates, 20 mg sodium per cup

- Light vanilla soymilk with 70 calories, 1.5 g fat, 6.0 g protein, 7.0 g carbohydrates (5 g sugar), 110 mg sodium per cup (such as Silk)

- Vanilla whey protein powder with 80 calories, 1.1 g fat, 16.0 g protein, 1.0 g carbohydrates, 65 mg sodium per 3/4 ounce

- Sugar substitute of your choice (I have used several different brands in creating the recipes.)

Blackberry Breeze Smoothie

*The flavors in this smoothie bring back fond memories of picking
wild blackberries along the side of rural roads in Normandy, France.
They only needed a touch of cinnamon to bring out their flavor.*

This smoothie can be made the night before and stored in the refrigerator.

Helpful Hints

- Use plain, frozen blackberries that are not in sugar syrup.
- Use a nonfat mixed-berry yogurt if blackberry is unavailable.

 1/2 cup frozen, unsweetened blackberries
 1/2 cup ripe banana, sliced
 1 cup nonfat blackberry yogurt
 1 scoop (3/4 ounce) vanilla whey protein powder
 1/4 teaspoon ground cinnamon
 2 tablespoons sliced almonds
 Sugar substitute equivalent to 2 teaspoons sugar

- Place frozen blackberries, banana, yogurt, whey protein powder, cinnamon, almonds, and sugar substitute in a blender.
- Blend 45 seconds or until smooth.

Makes one 16-ounce smoothie.

Exchanges/Food Choices: 1 1/2 fat-free milk, 3 carbohydrate, 2 lean protein
Per serving: Calories 370, Calories from Fat 70, Total Fat 8 g, Saturated Fat 1 g,
Trans Fat 0 g, Cholesterol 50 mg, Sodium 120 mg, Potassium 830 mg,
Total Carbohydrate 52 g, Dietary Fiber 8 g, Sugars 32 g, Protein 25 g, Phosphorus 245 mg

Shopping List:

1 small package frozen, unsweetened
   blackberries
1 ripe banana
1 carton nonfat blackberry yogurt
1 small package sliced almonds

Staples:

vanilla whey protein powder
ground cinnamon
sugar substitute

Shop Smart

- Nonfat vanilla or fruit-flavored yogurt with 140 calories, 16.0 g protein, 17.0 g carbohydrates, 75 mg sodium per 6-ounce carton
- Vanilla whey protein powder with 80 calories, 1.1 g fat, 16.0 g protein, 1.0 g carbohydrates, 65 mg sodium per 3/4 ounce
- Sugar substitute of your choice (I have used several different brands in creating the recipes.)

Blueberry Blast Smoothie

*Blueberries, full of healthy antioxidants, are one of my favorite
fruits. We used to pick them at a nearby farm in Connecticut
each summer. They were always big, juicy, and ripe.*

Helpful Hints

- Frozen, unsweetened blueberries can be used instead of fresh berries.
- Pasteurized, liquid egg whites can be found in cartons in the dairy/egg case.

3/4 cup blueberries
1 cup nonfat blueberry yogurt
1/2 cup pasteurized, liquid egg whites
Sugar substitute equivalent to 2 teaspoons sugar
1/2 teaspoon ground cinnamon
2 tablespoons sliced almonds
1 3/4 cups ice cubes

- Place blueberries, yogurt, egg whites, sugar substitute, cinnamon, and almonds in a blender.

- Blend about 30 seconds or until smooth.

- Add ice and blend 30 seconds or until thick.

Makes one 16-ounce smoothie.

*Exchanges/Food Choices: 2 fruit, 1 fat-free milk, 2 lean protein, 1 fat
Per serving: Calories 320, Calories from Fat 60, Total Fat 7 g, Saturated Fat 0.5 g,
Trans Fat 0 g, Cholesterol <5 mg, Sodium 320 mg, Potassium 680 mg,
Total Carbohydrate 45 g, Dietary Fiber 5 g, Sugars 30 g, Protein 23 g, Phosphorus 290 mg*

Shopping List:

1 small package blueberries
1 carton nonfat blueberry yogurt
1 small package sliced almonds

Staples:

pasteurized, liquid egg whites
sugar substitute
ground cinnamon

Shop Smart

- Pasteurized, liquid egg whites with 6 calories, 1.0 g fat, 1.0 g protein, 11 mg sodium per tablespoon
- Nonfat vanilla or fruit-flavored yogurt with 140 calories, 16.0 g protein, 17.0 g carbohydrates, 75 mg sodium per 6-ounce carton
- Sugar substitute of your choice (I have used several different brands in creating the recipes.)

Blueberry Green Tea Smoothie

This is a tasty smoothie packed with antioxidants.
It's best consumed as soon as it is made.

Helpful Hints

- Any type of green tea can be used.
- Firm tofu can be used instead of soft.
- Use plain, frozen blueberries that are not in sugar syrup.

1 green tea bag
1/2 cup boiling water
1 cup frozen, unsweetened blueberries
3/4 cup soft tofu
1/4 teaspoon ground cinnamon
1 scoop (3/4 ounce) vanilla whey protein powder
1 tablespoon dry-roasted cashew nuts without added salt
1 cup ice cubes

- Steep the tea bag in the water and let steep 4–5 minutes while assembling the other ingredients.

- Add blueberries, tofu, cinnamon, whey protein powder, and cashew nuts to a blender.

- Remove the tea bag from water and discard bag.

- Add tea to the blender and blend 30 seconds.

- Add the ice cubes and blend another 20 seconds or until smooth.

Makes one 16-ounce smoothie.

Exchanges/Food Choices: 1 fruit, 1 other carbohydrate, 4 lean protein
Per serving: Calories 330, Calories from Fat 25, Total Fat 13 g, Saturated Fat 2.5 g,
Trans Fat 0 g, Cholesterol 50 mg, Sodium 55 mg, Potassium 480 mg,
Total Carbohydrate 27 g, Dietary Fiber 5 g, Sugars 16 g, Protein 30 g, Phosphorus 230 mg

Shopping List:

1 container green tea bags
1 package frozen, unsweetened
   blueberries
1 package soft tofu
1 package dry-roasted cashew nuts
   without added salt

Staples:

ground cinnamon
vanilla whey protein powder

Shop Smart

- Soft tofu with 151 calories, 9.2 g fat, 16.2 g protein, 4.5 g carbohydrates, 20 mg sodium per cup
- Vanilla whey protein powder with 80 calories, 1.1 g fat, 16.0 g protein, 1.0 g carbohydrates, 65 mg sodium per 3/4 ounce

Cappuccino Smoothie

Capture the flavors of a good cup of cappuccino, coffee and frothy milk,
for your breakfast treat. A tasty biscotti completes your breakfast.

Helpful Hints

- Use powdered, instant regular or decaffeinated coffee. Do not mix it with water.
- Look for a biscotti with 100 calories, 5 g fat, 15 g carbohydrates, 75 mg sodium, such as Starbucks Vanilla Almond Biscotti.

    2 teaspoons instant espresso coffee
    1 cup fat-free milk
    1/2 cup pasteurized, liquid egg whites
    Sugar substitute equivalent to 2 teaspoons sugar
    1 biscotti (1 ounce)

- Place instant espresso coffee, milk, egg whites, and sugar substitute in a blender.
- Blend 30 seconds or until smooth.
- Serve with biscotti.

Makes one 12-ounce smoothie.

Exchanges/Food Choices: 1 starch, 1 fat-free milk, 2 lean protein
Per serving: Calories 260, Calories from Fat 20, Total Fat 2.5 g, Saturated Fat 0 g,
Trans Fat 0 g, Cholesterol 30 mg, Sodium 370 mg, Potassium 710 mg,
Total Carbohydrate 34 g, Dietary Fiber 1 g, Sugars 21 g, Protein 25 g, Phosphorus 275 mg

Shopping List:

1 small jar instant espresso
   coffee
1 small package biscotti

Staples:

fat-free milk
pasteurized, liquid egg whites
sugar substitute

Shop Smart

- Pasteurized, liquid egg whites with 6 calories, 1.0 g fat, 1.0 g protein, 11 mg sodium per tablespoon
- Biscotti with 100 calories, 5.0 g fat, 15.0 g carbohydrates, 75 mg sodium (such as Starbucks Vanilla Almond Biscotti)
- Sugar substitute of your choice (I have used several different brands in creating the recipes.)

Cherry Berry Smoothie

Sweet dark cherries and strawberries make a colorful and tasty combination in this simple smoothie. This smoothie can be made the night before and refrigerated until needed.

Helpful Hints

- Use a low-fat mixed-berry yogurt if cherry is not available.
- Use berries that are not packed in sugar syrup.

1/2 cup frozen, unsweetened, pitted cherries
1/2 cup frozen, unsweetened strawberries
1 cup low-fat cherry yogurt
1 scoop (3/4 ounce) vanilla whey protein powder

- Place cherries, strawberries, yogurt, and whey protein powder in a blender.

- Blend on high 1 minute or until smooth.

Makes one 13-ounce smoothie.

Exchanges/Food Choices: 1 fat-free milk, 2 1/2 carbohydrate, 2 lean protein
Per serving: Calories 360, Calories from Fat 40, Total Fat 4.5 g, Saturated Fat 2 g,
Trans Fat 0 g, Cholesterol 60 mg, Sodium 180 mg, Potassium 730 mg,
Total Carbohydrate 55 g, Dietary Fiber 3 g, Sugars 47 g, Protein 26 g, Phosphorus 300 mg

Shopping List:

1 package frozen, unsweetened, pitted cherries
1 package frozen, unsweetened strawberries
1 carton low-fat cherry yogurt

Staples:

vanilla whey protein powder

Shop Smart

- Low-fat vanilla or fruit-flavored yogurt (not fruit on the bottom) with 208 calories, 3.1 g fat, 12.1 g protein, 33.8 g carbohydrates, 162 mg sodium per cup
- Vanilla whey protein powder with 80 calories, 1.1 g fat, 16.0 g protein, 1.0 g carbohydrates, 65 mg sodium per 3/4 ounce

Citrus Smoothie

Wake up with this bright, sunny orange and pineapple smoothie.

Helpful Hints

- Be sure pineapple is ripe and sweet.
- For easy preparation, buy ready-to-eat orange segments and pineapple cubes in the produce department.

1 cup orange segments
1/2 cup fresh pineapple cubes
2 tablespoons toasted wheat germ
1/2 cup pasteurized, liquid egg whites
2 tablespoons unsalted walnuts
Sugar substitute equivalent to 2 teaspoons sugar

- Add orange segments, pineapple cubes, wheat germ, egg whites, walnuts, and sugar substitute to a blender.

- Blend 45 seconds or until smooth.

Makes one 16-ounce smoothie.

Exchanges/Food Choices: 3 fruit, 3 medium-fat protein
Per serving: Calories 340, Calories from Fat 100, Total Fat 12 g, Saturated Fat 1 g,
Trans Fat 0 g, Cholesterol 0 mg, Sodium 202 mg, Potassium 680 mg,
Total Carbohydrate 41 g, Dietary Fiber 8 g, Sugars 28 g, Protein 22 g, Phosphorus 245 mg

Shopping List:

1 container orange segments or 1 orange
1 container pineapple cubes
1 jar toasted wheat germ
1 package unsalted walnuts

Staples:

pasteurized, liquid egg whites
sugar substitute

Shop Smart

- Toasted wheat germ with 27 calories, 0.8 g fat, 2.0 g protein, 3.5 g carbohydrates, 0 mg sodium per tablespoon
- Pasteurized, liquid egg whites with 6 calories, 1.0 g fat, 1.0 g protein, 11 mg sodium per tablespoon
- Sugar substitute of your choice (I have used several different brands in creating the recipes.)

Coconut Pineapple Smoothie

This smoothie is like drinking a tropical breeze. Coconut and pineapple are flavors found in a piña colada. This is a bright, light smoothie.

Helpful Hints

- Any type of low-fat coconut-flavored yogurt can be used.
- Look for pineapple cubes in the produce section of the market.

1 cup low-fat coconut yogurt
1/2 cup fresh pineapple cubes
1/2 tablespoon desiccated coconut (sweetened flakes)
1/2 cup pasteurized, liquid egg whites
1 scoop (3/4 ounce) vanilla whey protein powder

- Add coconut yogurt, pineapple, desiccated coconut, egg whites, and whey protein powder to blender.

- Blend on high 45 seconds to 1 minute or until smooth.

Makes one 16-ounce smoothie.

Exchanges/Food Choices: 2 carbohydrate, 4 1/2 lean protein
Per serving: Calories 330, Calories from Fat 100, Total Fat 12 g, Saturated Fat 9 g,
Trans Fat 0 g, Cholesterol 50 mg, Sodium 130 mg, Potassium 360 mg,
Total Carbohydrate 35 g, Dietary Fiber 5 g, Sugars 27 g, Protein 23 g, Phosphorus 14 mg

Shopping List:

1 carton low-fat coconut yogurt
1 container fresh pineapple cubes
1 package desiccated coconut
  (sweetened flakes)

Staples:

pasteurized, liquid egg whites
vanilla whey protein powder

Shop Smart

- Low-fat vanilla or fruit-flavored yogurt (not fruit on the bottom) with 208 calories, 3.1 g fat, 12.1 g protein, 33.8 g carbohydrates, 162 mg sodium per cup
- Desiccated coconut flakes (sweetened) with 388 calories, 24.0 g fat, 44.1 g carbohydrates, 242 mg sodium per cup
- Pasteurized, liquid egg whites with 6 calories, 1.0 g fat, 1.0 g protein, 11 mg sodium per tablespoon
- Vanilla whey protein powder with 80 calories, 1.1 g fat, 16.0 g protein, 1.0 g carbohydrates, 65 mg sodium per 3/4 ounce

Mango Smoothie

I love the sweet flavor and soft texture of mangoes. They're one of the world's most popular fruits alongside bananas. When they're in season, late March through September, I cut the flesh into cubes and store them in the freezer. Frozen mango can be found in many supermarkets.

Helpful Hints

- If plain, low-fat mango yogurt isn't available, use a combination of mango and other fruit flavors.

1/2 cup mango cubes
1 cup low-fat mango-flavored yogurt
1/2 cup pasteurized, liquid egg whites
1 scoop (3/4 ounce) vanilla whey protein powder

- Add mango cubes, yogurt, egg whites, and whey protein powder to a blender.

- Blend on high 45 seconds to 1 minute or until smooth.

Makes one 16-ounce smoothie.

Exchanges/Food Choices: 1 fruit, 2 fat-free milk, 4 lean protein
Per serving: Calories 330, Calories from Fat 20, Total Fat 2 g, Saturated Fat 1 g,
Trans Fat 0 g, Cholesterol 50 mg, Sodium 350 mg, Potassium 790 mg,
Total Carbohydrate 40 g, Dietary Fiber 1 g, Sugars 32 g, Protein 37 g, Phosphorus 230 mg

Shopping List:

1 carton low-fat coconut yogurt
1 container fresh pineapple cubes
1 package desiccated coconut
  (sweetened flakes)

Staples:

pasteurized, liquid egg whites
vanilla whey protein powder

Shop Smart

- Low-fat vanilla or fruit-flavored yogurt (not fruit on the bottom) with 208 calories, 3.1 g fat, 12.1 g protein, 33.8 g carbohydrates, 162 mg sodium per cup

- Desiccated coconut flakes (sweetened) with 388 calories, 24.0 g fat, 44.1 g carbohydrates, 242 mg sodium per cup

- Pasteurized, liquid egg whites with 6 calories, 1.0 g fat, 1.0 g protein, 11 mg sodium per tablespoon

- Vanilla whey protein powder with 80 calories, 1.1 g fat, 16.0 g protein, 1.0 g carbohydrates, 65 mg sodium per 3/4 ounce

Mango Smoothie

I love the sweet flavor and soft texture of mangoes. They're one of the world's most popular fruits alongside bananas. When they're in season, late March through September, I cut the flesh into cubes and store them in the freezer. Frozen mango can be found in many supermarkets.

Helpful Hints

■ If plain, low-fat mango yogurt isn't available, use a combination of mango and other fruit flavors.

    1/2 cup mango cubes
    1 cup low-fat mango-flavored yogurt
    1/2 cup pasteurized, liquid egg whites
    1 scoop (3/4 ounce) vanilla whey protein powder

■ Add mango cubes, yogurt, egg whites, and whey protein powder to a blender.

■ Blend on high 45 seconds to 1 minute or until smooth.

Makes one 16-ounce smoothie.

Exchanges/Food Choices: 1 fruit, 2 fat-free milk, 4 lean protein
Per serving: Calories 330, Calories from Fat 20, Total Fat 2 g, Saturated Fat 1 g,
Trans Fat 0 g, Cholesterol 50 mg, Sodium 350 mg, Potassium 790 mg,
Total Carbohydrate 40 g, Dietary Fiber 1 g, Sugars 32 g, Protein 37 g, Phosphorus 230 mg

Shopping List:

1 container mango cubes
1 carton low-fat mango-flavored yogurt
   (8 ounces)

Staples:

pasteurized, liquid egg whites
vanilla whey protein powder

Shop Smart

- Low-fat vanilla or fruit-flavored yogurt (not fruit on the bottom) with 208 calories, 3.1 g fat, 12.1 g protein, 33.8 g carbohydrates, 162 mg sodium per cup
- Pasteurized, liquid egg whites with 6 calories, 1.0 g fat, 1.0 g protein, 11 mg sodium per tablespoon
- Vanilla whey protein powder with 80 calories, 1.1 g fat, 16.0 g protein, 1.0 g carbohydrates, 65 mg sodium per 3/4 ounce

Mocha Magic Smoothie

Chocolate and coffee blend together to make this a tasty, mocha treat.

Helpful Hints

- Look for a nonfat frozen yogurt without added sugar.
- Use powdered, instant regular or decaffeinated coffee. Do not mix it with water.

2 tablespoons cocoa powder, unsweetened
2 teaspoons instant espresso coffee
1/2 cup pasteurized, liquid egg whites
1 cup light chocolate-flavored soymilk
1/2 cup nonfat chocolate frozen yogurt without added sugar
1 tablespoon dry-roasted, unsalted peanuts
2 teaspoons sugar substitute
2 tablespoons ice cubes

- Add cocoa powder, instant espresso coffee, egg whites, soymilk, frozen yogurt, peanuts, and sugar substitute to a blender.
- Blend on high 30 seconds.
- Add ice cubes and blend 30 seconds or until smooth.

Makes one 16-ounce smoothie.

Exchanges/Food Choices: 1 fat-free milk, 2 carbohydrate, 2 lean protein
Per serving: Calories 400, Calories from Fat 90, Total Fat 10 g, Saturated Fat 2 g,
Trans Fat 0 g, Cholesterol < 5 mg, Sodium 390 mg, Potassium 1,210 mg,
Total Carbohydrate 51 g, Dietary Fiber 8 g, Sugars 30 g, Protein 27 g, Phosphorus 470 mg

Shopping List:

1 package unsweetened cocoa powder
1 small jar instant espresso coffee
1 carton light chocolate-flavored soymilk
1 container nonfat chocolate frozen yogurt
    without added sugar
1 package dry-roasted, unsalted peanuts

Staples:

pasteurized, liquid egg whites
sugar substitute

Shop Smart

- Pasteurized, liquid egg whites with 6 calories, 1.0 g fat, 1.0 g protein, 11 mg sodium per tablespoon
- Light chocolate-flavored soymilk with 90 calories, 1.5 g fat, 3.0 g protein, 16.0 g carbohydrates (14.0 g sugar), 85 mg sodium per cup
- Sugar substitute of your choice (I have used several different brands in creating the recipes.)

Nutty Peach Whip

Peaches give this smoothie a light, summery feel, while the walnuts add more flavor and texture. This smoothie can be made the night before and stored in the refrigerator.

Helpful Hints

- If you have time, heat the walnuts in a skillet or toaster oven to enhance their flavor.

1/2 cup frozen peach slices
1 cup low-fat peach-flavored yogurt
1/2 cup pasteurized, liquid egg whites
2 tablespoons unsalted walnuts

- Place peaches, yogurt, egg whites, and walnuts in a blender.

- Blend 1 minute or until smooth.

Makes one 16-ounce smoothie.

Exchanges/Food Choices: 1 fat-free milk, 2 1/2 carbohydrate, 2 lean protein, 1 fat
Per serving: Calories 430, Calories from Fat 120, Total Fat 13 g, Saturated Fat 3 g,
Trans Fat 0 g, Cholesterol 20 mg, Sodium 350 mg, Potassium 800 mg,
Total Carbohydrate 52 g, Dietary Fiber 2 g, Sugars 45 g, Protein 26 g, Phosphorus 350 mg

Shopping List:

1 package frozen peach slices
1 carton low-fat peach-flavored yogurt
1 small package unsalted walnuts

Staples:

pasteurized, liquid egg whites

Shop Smart

- Low-fat vanilla or fruit-flavored yogurt (not fruit on the bottom) with 208 calories, 3.1 g fat, 12.1 g protein, 33.8 g carbohydrates, 162 mg sodium per cup
- Pasteurized, liquid egg whites with 6 calories, 1.0 g fat, 1.0 g protein, 11 mg sodium per tablespoon

Oats and Almonds Smoothie

*Old-fashioned oats and a touch of maple syrup
make this a very modern, tasty smoothie.
Almonds add extra flavor and texture.*

Helpful Hints

- Any type of oats can be used.

1 cup nonfat vanilla yogurt
1/2 cup pasteurized, liquid egg whites
2 tablespoons sliced almonds
2 tablespoons old-fashioned oats
2 teaspoons maple syrup

- Add yogurt, egg whites, almonds, oats, and maple syrup to a blender.
- Blend on high 1 minute or until smooth.

Makes one 12-ounce smoothie.

*Exchanges/Food Choices: 1 1/2 fat-free milk, 3 carbohydrate, 2 lean protein
Per serving: Calories 450, Calories from Fat 100, Total Fat 11 g , Saturated
Fat 3 g, Trans Fat 0 g, Cholesterol 10 mg, Sodium 350 mg, Potassium 870 mg,
Total Carbohydrate 61 g, Dietary Fiber 3 g, Sugars 47 g, Protein 29 g, Phosphorus 460 mg*

Shopping List:

1 carton nonfat vanilla yogurt (8 ounces)
1 small package sliced almonds
1 small container old-fashioned oats
1 small bottle maple syrup

Staples:

pasteurized, liquid egg whites

Shop Smart

- Pasteurized, liquid egg whites with 6 calories, 1.0 g fat, 1.0 g protein, 11 mg sodium per tablespoon
- Nonfat vanilla or fruit-flavored yogurt with 140 calories, 16.0 g protein, 17.0 g carbohydrates, 75 mg sodium per 6-ounce carton

Passion Fruit Smoothie

Passion fruit is a delicious, tart, tropical fruit with flavors similar to a blend of pineapple, guava, and lime. You can make this smoothie in minutes using canned passion fruit nectar.

Helpful Hints

- Look for passion fruit nectar (such as Goya Passion Fruit). Frozen passion fruit pulp can be used.
- If passion fruit nectar isn't available, use pineapple juice. The flavor will be different but delicious.

1 cup nonfat vanilla yogurt
1/2 cup canned passion fruit nectar
1 scoop (3/4 ounce) vanilla whey protein powder
2 teaspoons honey

- Add yogurt, passion fruit, whey protein powder, and honey to a blender.

- Blend 30 seconds or until smooth.

Makes one 12-ounce smoothie.

Exchanges/Food Choices: 1 1/2 fat-free milk, 3 carbohydrate, 2 lean protein
Per serving: Calories 380, Calories from Fat 15, Total Fat 1.5 g, Saturated Fat 0.5 g, Trans Fat 0 g, Cholesterol 60 mg, Sodium 200 mg, Potassium 640 mg, Total Carbohydrate 67 g, Dietary Fiber <1 g, Sugars 59 g, Protein 25 g, Phosphorus 230 mg

Shopping List:

1 carton nonfat vanilla yogurt
1 can passion fruit nectar

Staples:

vanilla whey protein powder
honey

Shop Smart

- Nonfat vanilla or fruit-flavored yogurt with 140 calories, 16.0 g protein, 17.0 g carbohydrates, 75 mg sodium per 6-ounce carton
- Canned passion fruit nectar with 18.8 calories, 4.8 g carbohydrates per fluid ounce
- Vanilla whey protein powder with 80 calories, 1.1 g fat, 16.0 g protein, 1.0 g carbohydrates, 65 mg sodium per 3/4 ounce

Peanut Butter
Banana Smoothie

This smoothie is made with popular ingredients—peanut butter and bananas.

Helpful Hints

- Look for peanut butter without added sugar or salt.
- This smoothie can be made with fresh or frozen bananas.

> 1/2 cup ripe banana, sliced
> 1 1/2 tablespoons natural peanut butter, no sugar or salt added
> 1/4 cup dry, nonfat instant milk
> 1/2 cup pasteurized, liquid egg whites
> 1/2 cup fat-free milk
> Sugar substitute equal to 2 teaspoons sugar

- Add banana, peanut butter, instant milk, egg whites, fat-free milk, and sugar substitute to a blender.

- Blend on high 1 minute or until smooth.

Makes one 12-ounce smoothie.

Exchanges/Food Choices: 1 fruit, 1 1/2 fat-free milk, 3 lean protein, 3 fat
Per serving: Calories 370, Calories from Fat 120, Total Fat 13 g, Saturated Fat 2.5 g,
Trans Fat 0 g, Cholesterol 5 mg, Sodium 350 mg, Potassium 1100 mg,
Total Carbohydrate 39 g, Dietary Fiber 3 g, Sugars 27 g, Protein 30 g, Phosphorus 410 mg

Shopping List:

1 ripe banana
1 jar natural peanut butter, without added
　sugar or salt
1 package dry, nonfat instant milk

Staples:

pasteurized, liquid egg whites
fat-free milk
sugar substitute

Shop Smart

- Pasteurized, liquid egg whites with 6 calories, 1.0 g fat, 1.0 g protein, 11 mg sodium per tablespoon
- Sugar substitute of your choice (I have used several different brands in creating the recipes.)

Pear Cinnamon Smoothie

*Juicy ripe pears and cinnamon blend together
for this flavorful smoothie.*

Helpful Hints

■ Any type of ripe pear can be used.

> 1 cup low-fat vanilla yogurt
> 1/2 cup pasteurized, liquid egg whites
> 1/2 cup cubed ripe pear with skin
> 1/2 teaspoon ground cinnamon
> 2 tablespoons unsalted pecans

■ Place yogurt, egg whites, pear cubes, cinnamon, and pecans in a blender.

■ Blend on high 1 minute or until smooth.

Makes one 12-ounce smoothie.

*Exchanges/Food Choices: 1 fruit, 1 1/2 low-fat milk, 2 lean protein, 2 fat
Per serving: Calories 410, Calories from Fat 120, Total Fat 13 g, Saturated Fat 3 g,
Trans Fat 0 g, Cholesterol 10 mg, Sodium 360 mg, Potassium 890 mg,
Total Carbohydrate 50 g, Dietary Fiber 5 g, Sugars 43 g, Protein 27 g, Phosphorus 400 mg*

Shopping List: ## Staples:

1 carton low-fat vanilla yogurt (8 ounces)   pasteurized, liquid egg whites
1 ripe pear   ground cinnamon
1 package unsalted pecans

Shop Smart

■ Low-fat vanilla or fruit-flavored yogurt (not fruit on the bottom) with 208 calories, 3.1 g fat, 12.1 g protein, 33.8 g carbohydrates, 162 mg sodium per cup

■ Pasteurized, liquid egg whites with 6 calories, 1.0 g fat, 1.0 g protein, 11 mg sodium per tablespoon

Plum Perfect Smoothie

Dried plums, also called prunes, are soaked for a few minutes in milk before blending with the rest of the ingredients for this breakfast treat.

Helpful Hints
- This smoothie can be made a day ahead.

1/4 cup dried plums (prunes), pits removed
1/2 cup fat-free milk
6 tablespoons pasteurized, liquid egg whites
2/3 cup low-fat vanilla yogurt

- Place dried plums in the milk and let stand 15 minutes.
- Add to a blender with the milk, egg whites, and yogurt.
- Blend on high for 1 minute or until smooth.

Makes one 18-ounce smoothie.

Exchanges/Food Choices: 2 fruit, 1 1/2 low-fat milk, 1 1/2 lean protein
Per serving: Calories 330, Calories from Fat 20, Total Fat 2.5 g, Saturated Fat 1.5 g, Trans Fat 0 g, Cholesterol 10 mg, Sodium 310 mg, Potassium 1010 mg, Total Carbohydrate 56 g, Dietary Fiber 3 g, Sugars 46 g, Protein 23 g, Phosphorus 390 mg

Shopping List:
1 package dried plums (prunes), pits removed
1 carton low-fat vanilla yogurt

Staples:
fat-free milk
pasteurized, liquid egg whites

Shop Smart
- Pasteurized, liquid egg whites with 6 calories, 1.0 g fat, 1.0 g protein, 11 mg sodium per tablespoon
- Low-fat vanilla or fruit-flavored yogurt (not fruit on the bottom) with 208 calories, 3.1 g fat, 12.1 g protein, 33.8 g carbohydrates, 162 mg sodium per cup

Strawberry Almond Smoothie

Almonds and dried cranberries add flavor
to sweet strawberries for this smoothie.

Helpful Hints

- Slivered almonds can be used instead of sliced almonds.
- Firm tofu can be used instead of soft.

> 1 cup frozen, unsweetened strawberries
> 3 tablespoons dried cranberries
> 2 tablespoons sliced almonds
> 1/2 cup plain soft tofu
> 1/2 teaspoon almond extract
> 1/2 cup pasteurized, liquid egg whites
> Sugar substitute equivalent to 2 teaspoons sugar

- Add strawberries, cranberries, almonds, tofu, almond extract, egg whites, and sugar substitute in a blender.

- Blend on high 1 minute or until smooth.

Makes one 10-ounce smoothie.

Exchanges/Food Choices: 2 fruit, 1/2 other carbohydrate, 3 lean protein, 2 fat
Per serving: Calories 365, Calories from Fat 100, Total Fat 11 g, Saturated Fat 1 g,
Trans Fat 0 g, Cholesterol 0 mg, Sodium 220 mg, Potassium 760 mg,
Total Carbohydrate 48 g, Dietary Fiber 7 g, Sugars 27 g, Protein 25 g, Phosphorus 220 mg

Shopping List:

1 package frozen, unsweetened
    strawberries
1 package dried cranberries
1 small package sliced almonds
1 small package plain soft tofu
1 bottle almond extract

Staples:

pasteurized, liquid egg whites
sugar substitute

Shop Smart

- Soft tofu with 151 calories, 9.2 g fat, 16.2 g protein, 4.5 g carbohydrates, 20 mg sodium per cup
- Pasteurized, liquid egg whites with 6 calories, 1.0 g fat, 1.0 g protein, 11 mg sodium per tablespoon
- Sugar substitute of your choice (I have used several different brands in creating the recipes.)

Virgin Bloody Mary Smoothie

Wake up your taste buds with this spicy smoothie that has a rich, tomato flavor.

Helpful Hints

- Firm tofu can be used instead of soft.

> 3/4 cup low-sodium tomato juice
> 1/2 cup sun-dried tomatoes packed in oil, well drained
> 1 teaspoon horseradish
> Several drops Worcestershire sauce
> 1/4 cup soft tofu
> 1 scoop (3/4 ounce) vanilla whey protein powder
> 1 small piece light creamy Swiss cheese (3/4 ounce) (similar to Laughing Cow Wedges)
> 1 slice whole-wheat toast

- Place tomato juice, sun-dried tomatoes, horseradish, Worcestershire sauce, tofu, and whey protein powder in a blender.

- Blend 30 seconds or until smooth.

- Serve with whole-wheat toast spread with the creamy Swiss cheese.

Makes one 16-ounce smoothie.

Exchanges/Food Choices: 2 starch, 2 vegetable, 2 medium-fat protein, 1 fat
Per serving: Calories 400, Calories from Fat 140, Total Fat 14 g, Saturated Fat 3 g,
Trans Fat 0 g, Cholesterol 50 mg, Sodium 550 mg, Potassium 1500 mg,
Total Carbohydrate 40 g, Dietary Fiber 8 g, Sugars 10 g, Protein 30 g, Phosphorus 245 mg

Shopping List:

- 1 can low-sodium tomato juice (6 ounces)
- 1 package sundried tomatoes packed in oil
- 1 bottle horseradish
- 1 bottle Worcestershire sauce
- 1 package soft tofu
- 1 package light creamy Swiss cheese (3/4 ounce) (similar to Laughing Cow Wedges)

Staples:

vanilla whey protein powder
whole-wheat bread

Shop Smart

- Low-sodium tomato juice with 41 calories, 10.3 g carbohydrates, 24 mg sodium per cup
- Soft tofu with 151 calories, 9.2 g fat, 16.2 g protein, 4.5 g carbohydrates, 20 mg sodium per cup
- Vanilla whey protein powder with 80 calories, 1.1 g fat, 16.0 g protein, 1.0 g carbohydrates, 65 mg sodium per 3/4 ounce
- Swiss cheese (such as light Laughing Cow Wedges) with 35 calories, 2.0 g fat, 2.5 g protein, 260 mg sodium for 3/4 ounce piece

Raspberry Wakeup Smoothie

*Raspberries, packed with flavor and fiber, combine
with walnuts for this tasty, nutty smoothie.*

Helpful Hints

- If raspberry yogurt isn't available, use a mixed-berry yogurt.

  3/4 cup low-fat raspberry yogurt
  1/2 cup frozen, unsweetened raspberries
  1/3 cup dry, nonfat instant powdered milk
  2 tablespoons unsalted walnuts
  1/4 cup fat-free milk

- Add yogurt, raspberries, instant powdered milk, walnuts, and fat-free milk to
  a blender.

- Blend on high 1 minute or until smooth.

Makes one 10-ounce smoothie.

*Exchanges/Food Choices: 1 fruit, 2 fat-free milk, 2 1/2 fat
Per serving: Calories 410, Calories from Fat 120, Total Fat 13 g, Saturated Fat 2.5 g,
Trans Fat 0 g, Cholesterol 20 mg, Sodium 260 mg, Potassium 930 mg,
Total Carbohydrate 55 g, Dietary Fiber 5 g, Sugars 46 g, Protein 20 g, Phosphorus 555 mg.*

Shopping List:

1 carton low-fat raspberry yogurt
   (6 ounces)
1 package frozen, unsweetened
   raspberries
1 package dry, nonfat instant powdered
   milk
1 package unsalted walnuts

Staples:

fat-free milk

Shop Smart

- Low-fat vanilla or fruit-flavored yogurt (not fruit on the bottom) with 208
  calories, 3.1 g fat, 12.1 g protein, 33.8 g carbohydrates, 162 mg sodium per cup

Lunch

Banana Sunbutter Shake

Sunbutter is made from sunflower seeds and is rich in protein. It makes a nutty, thick lunch shake.

Helpful Hints

- Sunbutter can be found in most supermarkets.
- Look for light almond milk with no sugar added.

1 cup ripe banana, sliced
2 tablespoons creamy sunbutter
1/2 cup light, unsweetened almond milk
1 scoop (3/4 ounce) vanilla whey protein powder

- Add banana, sunbutter, almond milk, and whey protein powder to a blender.
- Blend 45 seconds or until smooth.

Makes one 8-ounce smoothie.

Exchanges/Food Choices: 3 fruit, 4 medium-fat protein
Per serving: Calories 460, Calories from Fat 200, Total Fat 22 g, Saturated Fat 2.5 g,
Trans Fat 0 g, Cholesterol 50 mg, Sodium 50 mg, Potassium 990 mg,
Total Carbohydrate 46 g, Dietary Fiber 8 g, Sugars 23 g, Protein 28 g, Phosphorus 245 mg

Shopping List:

1 ripe banana
1 jar creamy sunbutter
1 carton light, unsweetened almond milk

Staples:

vanilla whey protein powder

Shop Smart

- Sunbutter with 100 calories, 8.0 g fat, 3.5 g protein, 3.5 carbohydrates, 60 mg sodium per tablespoon
- Unsweetened almond milk with 3.0 g fat and 2.0 g carbohydrates per cup
- Vanilla whey protein powder with 80 calories, 1.1 g fat, 16.0 g protein, 1.0 g carbohydrates, 65 mg sodium per 3/4 ounce

Beets and Cream Borscht Smoothie

Borscht, a soup made with beets, can be served hot or cold and is always garnished with a dollop of sour cream. This smoothie captures the flavors of this Russian dish, including the dollop of sour cream.

Helpful Hints

- Buy canned beets that do not have added sugar.

1 1/2 cups canned beets, not packed in sugar, rinsed, drained, and sliced
2 tablespoons nonfat sour cream
1/2 cup pasteurized, liquid egg whites
1 scoop (3/4 ounce) vanilla whey protein powder
1/2 cup canned or bottled carrot juice
1 teaspoon olive oil
1/4 cup sliced onion
Salt and freshly ground black pepper

- Place beets, sour cream, egg whites, whey protein powder, carrot juice, olive oil, and onion in a blender.

- Add salt and pepper to taste.

- Blend 30 seconds or until smooth.

Makes one 20-ounce smoothie.

Exchanges/Food Choices: 3 fruit, 5 lean protein
Per serving: Calories 380, Calories from Fat 60, Total Fat 7 g, Saturated Fat 1.5 g, Trans Fat 0 g, Cholesterol 40 mg, Sodium 420 mg, Potassium 1300 mg, Total Carbohydrate 45 g, Dietary Fiber 6 g, Sugars 30 g, Protein 35 g, Phosphorus 170 mg

Shopping List:

1 jar or can sliced beets (not packed in sugar)

1 carton nonfat sour cream

1 small can or bottle carrot juice

Staples:

pasteurized, liquid egg whites

vanilla whey protein powder

olive oil

onion

salt and black peppercorns

Shop Smart

- Pasteurized, liquid egg whites with 6 calories, 1.0 g fat, 1.0 g protein, 11 mg sodium per tablespoon
- Nonfat sour cream with 9 calories, 0.4 g protein, 1.9 g carbohydrates, 17 mg sodium per tablespoon
- Vanilla whey protein powder with 80 calories, 1.1 g fat, 16.0 g protein, 1.0 g carbohydrates, 65 mg sodium per 3/4 ounce
- Carrot juice with 94 calories, 21.9 g carbohydrates, 156 mg sodium per cup

Cantaloupe Crush Smoothie

Sweet, ripe cantaloupe melon gives this smoothie a delicate, melon flavor. To tell whether a cantaloupe is ripe, press the stem end. It should give a little. Another sign is if it smells sweet and ready to eat.

Helpful Hints

- Cantaloupe cubes can be found in the produce section of the supermarket. These precut cubes are usually ripe and ready to eat.

1/2 cup light vanilla soymilk (such as Silk)
1 cup low-fat vanilla yogurt
1 cup ripe cantaloupe, cubed
1/2 cup pasteurized, liquid egg whites
1 teaspoon vanilla extract
Sugar substitute equivalent to 2 teaspoons sugar
2 tablespoons sliced almonds

- Place soymilk, yogurt, cantaloupe cubes, egg whites, vanilla extract, sugar substitute, and almonds in a blender.

- Blend 45 seconds or until smooth.

Makes one 18-ounce smoothie.

Exchanges/Food Choices: 1 fruit, 1 1/2 fat-free milk, 2 lean protein, 2 fat
Per serving: Calories 450, Calories from Fat 90, Total Fat 10 g, Saturated Fat 2.5 g, Trans Fat 0 g, Cholesterol 10 mg, Sodium 470 mg, Potassium 1390 mg, Total Carbohydrate 57 g, Dietary Fiber 4 g, Sugars 49 g, Protein 32 g, Phosphorus 554 mg

1 small container light vanilla soymilk

1 carton low-fat vanilla yogurt

1 small container ripe cantaloupe cubes

1 small package sliced almonds

pasteurized, liquid egg whites

vanilla extract

sugar substitute

Shop Smart

- Light vanilla soymilk with 70 calories, 1.5 g fat, 6.0 g protein, 7.0 g carbohydrates (5 g sugar), 110 mg sodium per cup (such as Silk)

- Low-fat vanilla or fruit-flavored yogurt (not fruit on the bottom) with 208 calories, 3.1 g fat, 12.1 g protein, 33.8 g carbohydrates, 162 mg sodium per cup

- Pasteurized, liquid egg whites with 6 calories, 1.0 g fat, 1.0 g protein, 11 mg sodium per tablespoon

- Sugar substitute of your choice (I have used several different brands in creating the recipes.)

Carrot, Ginger, and Orange Smoothie

Fresh ginger brightens this carrot- and orange-flavored smoothie.

Helpful Hints

- Buy sliced carrots in the produce section of the market.
- A quick way to peel ginger is to scrape the skin off with the edge of a spoon.

> 1 teaspoon fresh ginger, cut into small pieces
> 1 cup sliced carrots
> 1/2 cup orange juice
> 1 scoop (3/4 ounce) vanilla whey protein powder
> 1/2 cup pasteurized, liquid egg whites
> 1/4 cup nonfat ricotta cheese, no salt added

- Peel ginger and cut into small pieces to measure 1 teaspoon full.

- Place ginger in a blender with the carrots, orange juice, whey protein powder, egg whites, and ricotta cheese.

- Blend 45 seconds or until smooth.

Makes one 14-ounce smoothie.

Exchanges/Food Choices: 2 fruit, 3 vegetable, 5 lean protein
Per serving: Calories 360, Calories from Fat 25, Total Fat 2.5 g, Saturated Fat 1 g,
Trans Fat 0 g, Cholesterol 60 mg, Sodium 460 mg, Potassium 1320 mg,
Total Carbohydrate 45 g, Dietary Fiber 5 g, Sugars 33 g, Protein 39 g, Phosphorus 220 mg

Shopping List:

1 small piece fresh ginger
1 package sliced carrots
1 small bottle orange juice (4 ounces)
1 small container nonfat ricotta cheese,
   no salt added

Staples:

vanilla whey protein powder
pasteurized, liquid egg whites

Shop Smart

- Vanilla whey protein powder with 80 calories, 1.1 g fat, 16.0 g protein, 1.0 g carbohydrates, 65 mg sodium per 3/4 ounce
- Pasteurized, liquid egg whites with 6 calories, 1.0 g fat, 1.0 g protein, 11 mg sodium per tablespoon
- Nonfat ricotta cheese with 200 calories, 20.0 g protein, 20.0 g carbohydrates, 260 mg sodium per cup

Curried Gazpacho Smoothie

Fresh tomatoes and celery combine with curry powder to make this a gazpacho smoothie with an Indian twist.

Helpful Hints

- Mild and hot curry powder can be found in the spice section of the supermarket. This recipe calls for mild. If you like your drinks hot and spicy use the stronger curry powder. Make sure your curry powder is less than 3 months old. It loses its flavor after that time.
- Toasted wheat germ gives a slightly nutty flavor. Regular wheat germ can be used.

1/2 cup low-sodium tomato juice
1/2 cup tomato cubes
1/2 cup sliced celery
1 teaspoon mild curry powder
1/2 cup pasteurized, liquid egg whites
1 teaspoon olive oil
2 teaspoons balsamic vinegar
1/4 cup toasted wheat germ
1 ounce lean, low-sodium sliced turkey breast
1 slice whole-wheat toast

- Place tomato juice, tomatoes, celery, curry powder, egg whites, olive oil, vinegar, and wheat germ in a blender.

- Blend 30 seconds or until smooth.

- Place turkey on bread and serve with smoothie.

Makes one 12-ounce smoothie.

Exchanges/Food Choices: 2 1/2 starch, 2 vegetable, 4 lean protein, 1 fat
Per serving: Calories 367, Calories from Fat 90, Total Fat 9.5 g, Saturated Fat 1.5 g,
Trans Fat 0 g, Cholesterol 15 mg, Sodium 655 mg, Potassium 1210 mg,
Total Carbohydrate 39 g, Dietary Fiber 10 g, Sugars 15 g, Protein 33 g, Phosphorus 500 mg

Shopping List:

1 bottle low-sodium tomato juice
1 tomato
1 small bunch celery
1 bottle mild curry powder
1 jar toasted wheat germ
1 ounce lean, low-sodium turkey breast

Staples:

pasteurized, liquid egg whites
olive oil
balsamic vinegar
whole-wheat bread

Shop Smart

- Low-sodium tomato juice with 41 calories, 10.3 g carbohydrates, 24 mg sodium per cup
- Pasteurized, liquid egg whites with 6 calories, 1.0 g fat, 1.0 g protein, 11 mg sodium per tablespoon
- Toasted wheat germ with 27 calories, 0.8 g fat, 2.0 g protein, 3.5 g carbohydrates, 0 mg sodium per tablespoon

Cherry Egg Cream Smoothie

Egg cream is a popular New York drink that doesn't have eggs. It's traditionally made from chocolate syrup, milk, and seltzer. This smoothie uses cherries instead of chocolate reducing the calories and the fat.

Helpful Hints

- Look for frozen, sweet cherries not in sugar syrup.
- Any type of low-fat cherry-flavored yogurt can be used.

> 1 cup frozen, unsweetened, pitted cherries
> 1 cup nonfat cherry yogurt
> 1 teaspoon olive oil
> 1 scoop (3/4 ounce) vanilla whey protein powder
> 1/2 cup sparkling water

- Place cherries, yogurt, olive oil, whey protein powder, and sparkling water in a blender.
- Blend 45 seconds or until smooth.

Makes one 16-ounce smoothie.

Exchanges/Food Choices: 1 fat-free milk, 3 1/2 carbohydrate, 2 lean protein
Per serving: Calories 310, Calories from Fat 60, Total Fat 7 g, Saturated Fat 1.5 g,
Trans Fat 0 g, Cholesterol 50 mg, Sodium 150 mg, Potassium 640 mg,
Total Carbohydrate 42 g, Dietary Fiber 3 g, Sugars 31 g, Protein 25 g, Phosphorus 240 mg

Shopping List:

1 small package frozen, unsweetened, pitted cherries
1 carton nonfat cherry yogurt
1 small bottle sparkling water

Staples:

olive oil
vanilla whey protein powder

Shop Smart

- Nonfat vanilla or fruit-flavored yogurt with 140 calories, 16.0 g protein, 17.0 g carbohydrates, 75 mg sodium per 6-ounce carton
- Vanilla whey protein powder with 80 calories, 1.1 g fat, 16.0 g protein, 1.0 g carbohydrates, 65 mg sodium per 3/4 ounce

Mango Lassi Smoothie

Freshly picked mangos, still warm from the sun, mixed with plain yogurt is a thirst-quenching Indian specialty. This smoothie captures the essence of this drink.

Helpful Hints

■ Ripe, fresh mangoes work best for this drink. Frozen mango pulp found in some supermarkets also works well.

> 1 cup nonfat plain yogurt
> 3/4 cup ripe mango, cubed, or frozen mango pulp
> 1/2 cup pasteurized, liquid egg whites
> Sugar substitute equivalent to 2 teaspoons sugar
> 1/2 teaspoon vanilla extract
> 2 tablespoons shelled pistachio nuts, dry roasted without salt added

■ Place yogurt, mango, egg whites, sugar substitute, vanilla extract, and pistachios in a blender.

■ Blend 20–30 seconds or until smooth.

Makes one 16-ounce smoothie.

Exchanges/Food Choices: 1 1/2 fruit, 1 1/2 low-fat milk, 3 lean protein, 1 fat
Per serving: Calories 370, Calories from Fat 70, Total Fat 8 g, Saturated Fat 1 g,
Trans Fat 0 g, Cholesterol <5 mg , Sodium 390 mg, Potassium 1190 mg,
Total Carbohydrate 44 g, Dietary Fiber 4 g, Sugars 38 g, Protein 32 g, Phosphorus 490 mg

Shopping List:

1 small container nonfat plain yogurt
1 small, ripe mango or frozen mango pulp
1 small package shelled pistachio nuts,
 dry roasted without salt

Staples:

pasteurized, liquid egg whites
vanilla extract
sugar substitute

Shop Smart

■ Nonfat yogurt with 103 calories, 4.0 g fat, 9.3 g protein, 18.1 g carbohydrates, 142 mg sodium per cup

■ Pasteurized, liquid egg whites with 6 calories, 1.0 g fat, 1.0 g protein, 11 mg sodium per tablespoon

■ Sugar substitute of your choice (I have used several different brands in creating the recipes.)

Mississippi Mud Pie Smoothie

Chocolate, cream, and pecans are ingredients for this popular Southern dessert. This smoothie captures the essence of the pie without the guilty calories.

Helpful Hints

- This smoothie is best when served immediately.

    1 1/2 tablespoons nonfat sour cream
    1 cup nonfat vanilla yogurt
    1/2 cup pasteurized, liquid egg whites
    2 teaspoons cocoa powder, unsweetened
    1/2 cup light, chocolate-flavored soymilk (such as Silk)
    2 tablespoons unsalted pecan pieces
    2 graham crackers (2 1/2 inches square each)

- Place sour cream, yogurt, egg whites, cocoa powder, soymilk, and pecans in a blender.

- Blend 30 seconds or until smooth.

- Serve with the graham crackers.

Makes one 16-ounce smoothie.

Exchanges/Food Choices: 2 starch, 1 low-fat milk, 2 medium fat protein, 1 fat
Per serving: Calories 460, Calories from Fat 120, Total Fat 13 g, Saturated Fat 1.5 g,
Trans Fat 0 g, Cholesterol <5 mg, Sodium 510 mg, Potassium 530 mg,
Total Carbohydrate 59 g, Dietary Fiber 4 g, Sugars 45 g, Protein 29 g, Phosphorus 225 mg

Shopping List:

1 container nonfat sour cream
1 container nonfat vanilla yogurt
1 package unsweetened cocoa powder
1 carton light chocolate-flavored soymilk
1 package unsalted pecan pieces
1 small box graham crackers

Staples:

pasteurized, liquid egg whites

Shop Smart

- Nonfat sour cream with 9 calories, 0.4 g protein, 1.9 g carbohydrates, 17 mg sodium per tablespoon
- Nonfat vanilla or fruit-flavored yogurt with 140 calories, 16.0 g protein, 17.0 g carbohydrates, 75 mg sodium per 6-ounce carton
- Pasteurized, liquid egg whites with 6 calories, 1.0 g fat, 1.0 g protein, 11 mg sodium per tablespoon
- Light chocolate-flavored soymilk with 90 calories, 1.5 g fat, 3.0 g protein, 16.0 g carbohydrates (14.0 g sugar), 85 mg sodium per cup (such as Silk)

Mocha Mint Smoothie

Fresh mint adds a bright touch to this rich, chocolate- and coffee-flavored smoothie. Serve it with some ripe, sliced bananas on the side.

Helpful Hints

- Use powdered, instant regular or decaffeinated coffee for the recipe. Do not mix it with water.

1 tablespoon cocoa powder, unsweetened
1 cup low-fat vanilla yogurt
1 teaspoon instant coffee powder
1/2 cup pasteurized, liquid egg whites
1 teaspoon canola oil
1/2 cup fresh mint leaves
1/2 cup ripe banana, sliced

- Place cocoa powder, yogurt, instant coffee, egg whites, canola oil, and mint in a blender.

- Blend 34–40 seconds or until smooth.

- Serve sliced bananas in a small bowl on the side.

Makes one 8-ounce smoothie.

Exchanges/Food Choices: 1 1/2 fat-free milk, 1 1/2 carbohydrate, 2 lean protein
Per serving: Calories 340, Calories from Fat 80, Total Fat 8.5 g, Saturated Fat 3 g,
Trans Fat 0 g, Cholesterol 10 mg, Sodium 370 mg, Potassium 750 mg,
Total Carbohydrate 40 g, Dietary Fiber 3 g, Sugars 34 g, Protein 27 g, Phosphorus 385 mg

Shopping List:

1 package unsweetened cocoa powder
1 carton low-fat vanilla yogurt
1 jar instant coffee powder
1 ripe banana
1 bunch fresh mint

Staples:

pasteurized, liquid egg whites
canola oil

Shop Smart

- Low-fat vanilla or fruit-flavored yogurt (not fruit on the bottom) with 208 calories, 3.1 g fat, 12.1 g protein, 33.8 g carbohydrates, 162 mg sodium per cup
- Pasteurized, liquid egg whites with 6 calories, 1.0 g fat, 1.0 g protein, 11 mg sodium per tablespoon

Nutty Butter Blizzard Smoothie (Peanut Butter Smoothie)

This thick smoothie is packed with a nutty, peanut butter flavor.
It can be made a day ahead and stored in the refrigerator.

Helpful Hints

- Look for peanut butter without added sugar or salt.
- Any flavor low-sugar jam or jelly can be used.

> 1 1/2 tablespoons crunchy natural peanut butter, without added salt or sugar
> 1 tablespoon low-sugar grape jam
> 1/2 cup nonfat ricotta cheese, no salt added
> 1/2 cup pasteurized, liquid egg whites
> 1/2 teaspoon almond extract

- Place peanut butter, grape jam, ricotta cheese, egg whites, and almond extract in a blender.

- Blend 30 seconds or until smooth.

Makes one 12-ounce smoothie.

Exchanges/Food Choices: 1 carbohydrate, 4 lean protein, 2 fat
Per serving: Calories 320, Calories from Fat 110, Total Fat 12 g, Saturated Fat 2.5 g,
Trans Fat 0 g, Cholesterol 30 mg, Sodium 510 mg, Potassium 370 mg,
Total Carbohydrate 21 g, Dietary Fiber 2 g, Sugars 18 g, Protein 31 g, Phosphorus 105 mg

Shopping List:

1 jar crunchy natural peanut butter, without added salt or sugar
1 small jar low-sugar grape jam
1 carton nonfat ricotta cheese, no salt added
1 bottle almond extract

Staples:

pasteurized, liquid egg whites

Shop Smart

- Low-sugar grape jam with 56 calories, 13.8 g carbohydrates per tablespoon
- Nonfat ricotta cheese with 200 calories, 20.0 g protein, 20.0 g carbohydrates, 260 mg sodium per cup
- Pasteurized, liquid egg whites with 6 calories, 1.0 g fat, 1.0 g protein, 11 mg sodium per tablespoon

Orange-Kiwi Whip

*Toasted walnuts add an intriguing flavor to kiwis and
orange juice for this colorful smoothie.*

Helpful Hints

- Look for ripe kiwis. They should give slightly when pressed with your thumb.
- To quickly remove the kiwi flesh, cut it in half lengthwise and scoop the flesh out with a spoon.

> 2 tablespoons unsalted walnuts
> 1/2 cup sliced kiwi fruit
> 1/2 cup orange juice
> 1/2 tablespoon honey
> 1 scoop (3/4 ounce) vanilla whey protein powder
> 1/2 cup ice cubes

- Place walnuts on a baking tray and toast in a toaster oven or under the broiler for 1–2 minutes or until slightly brown.
- Add walnuts to a blender with the kiwi, orange juice, honey, and whey protein powder.
- Blend 30 seconds.
- Add ice cubes and blend 30 seconds or until smooth.

Makes one 12-ounce smoothie.

*Exchanges/Food Choices: 2 fruit, 1/2 carbohydrate, 3 lean protein, 1/2 fat
Per serving: Calories 330, Calories from Fat 100, Total Fat 11 g, Saturated Fat 1.5 g,
Trans Fat 0 g, Cholesterol 50 mg, Sodium 40 mg, Potassium 670 mg,
Total Carbohydrate 38 g, Dietary Fiber 3 g, Sugars 30 g, Protein 20 g, Phosphorus 50 mg*

Shopping List:

1 small package unsalted walnuts
2 ripe kiwi fruit
1 small carton or bottle orange juice

Staples:

honey
vanilla whey protein powder

Shop Smart

- Vanilla whey protein powder with 80 calories, 1.1 g fat, 16.0 g protein, 1.0 g carbohydrates, 65 mg sodium per 3/4 ounce

Pear Avocado Passion Smoothie

The blend of ripe avocado and sweet pear makes a delicate, thick, creamy smoothie. It should be enjoyed as soon as it is made.

Helpful Hints

- To speed ripening of the avocado and pear, remove stem from avocado and place both in a paper bag and leave in a warm spot.
- Toasted wheat germ gives a slightly nutty flavor. Regular wheat germ can be used.

> 1/2 cup ripe California (Hass-type) avocado, cubed
> 3/4 cup ripe pear, with skin, cubed
> 1/2 cup pasteurized, liquid egg whites
> 1/4 cup toasted wheat germ
> 1 scoop (3/4 ounce) vanilla whey protein powder

- Place avocado cubes, pear cubes, egg whites, wheat germ, and whey protein powder in a blender.

- Blend for 30 seconds or until smooth.

Makes one 10-ounce smoothie.

Exchanges/Food Choices: 1 starch, 1 1/2 fruit, 5 lean protein, 1 fat
Per serving: Calories 450, Calories from Fat 240, Total Fat 16 g, Saturated Fat 3 g,
Trans Fat 0 g, Cholesterol 50 mg, Sodium 240 mg, Potassium 890 mg,
Total Carbohydrate 41 g, Dietary Fiber 13 g, Sugars 16 g, Protein 40 g, Phosphorus 375 mg

Shopping List:

1 ripe, California (Hass-type) avocado
1 ripe pear
1 jar toasted wheat germ

Staples:

pasteurized, liquid egg whites
vanilla whey protein powder

Shop Smart

- Pasteurized, liquid egg whites with 6 calories, 1.0 g fat, 1.0 g protein, 11 mg sodium per tablespoon
- Toasted wheat germ with 27 calories, 0.8 g fat, 2.0 g protein, 3.5 g carbohydrates, 0 mg sodium per tablespoon
- Vanilla whey protein powder with 80 calories, 1.1 g fat, 16.0 g protein, 1.0 g carbohydrates, 65 mg sodium per 3/4 ounce

Pesto Pizzazz Smoothie

Pesto sauce made with fresh basil, parsley, pine nuts, and Parmesan cheese is available ready prepared in most markets. Combined with ricotta cheese, it makes a tasty smoothie that can be used for a quick meal on the go. Add a slice of Parmesan toast to complete this lunch.

Helpful Hints

- This smoothie should be eaten immediately or, place the ingredients in a blender jar and store in the refrigerator. When needed, simply place the jar on the blender and process.
- Look for a prepared low-fat pesto sauce (such as Buitoni).

> 1 tablespoon prepared, reduced-fat pesto sauce (such as Buitoni)
> 1/2 cup nonfat ricotta cheese
> 1/2 cup fat-free, low-sodium chicken broth
> 3 tablespoons cracker meal
> 1 slice whole-wheat bread (1 ounce)
> 2 tablespoons grated Parmesan cheese

- Add pesto sauce, ricotta cheese, chicken broth, and cracker meal to a blender.

- Blend 35–40 seconds.

- Sprinkle bread with grated Parmesan cheese and place in a toaster oven or under the broiler for about 30 seconds or until the cheese starts to melt.

- Serve Parmesan toast with the smoothie.

Makes one 8-ounce smoothie.

Exchanges/Food Choices: 2 1/2 starch, 2 lean protein, 1 fat
Per serving: Calories 360, Calories from Fat 90, Total Fat 9.5 g, Saturated Fat 3 g,
Trans Fat 0 g, Cholesterol 40 mg, Sodium 570 mg, Potassium 510 mg,
Total Carbohydrate 39 g, Dietary Fiber 3 g, Sugars 9 g, Protein 26 g, Phosphorus 410 mg

Shopping List:

1 container reduced-fat, pesto sauce
  (such as Buitoni)
1 small carton nonfat ricotta cheese
1 box cracker meal
1 small piece Parmesan cheese

Staples:

fat-free, low-sodium chicken broth
whole-wheat bread

Shop Smart

- Nonfat ricotta cheese with 200 calories, 20.0 g protein, 20.0 g carbohydrates, 260 mg sodium per cup
- Cracker meal with 440 calories, 2.0 g fat, 10.7 g protein, 93.0 g carbohydrates, 18 g sodium per cup

Pomegranate Smoothie

The tangy flavor of pomegranate is brought out in this tart and sweet smoothie. Flaxseed meal adds a nutty flavor.

Helpful Hints

- Ground flaxseed can be used instead of flaxseed meal.
- Store flaxseed in the refrigerator to keep it from becoming rancid.

1/2 cup 100% pomegranate juice, unsweetened
1/2 cup light vanilla soymilk
1 cup low-fat vanilla yogurt
1 scoop (3/4 ounce) vanilla whey protein powder
1 tablespoon flaxseed meal
Sugar substitute equivalent to 2 teaspoons sugar

- Place pomegranate juice, soymilk, yogurt, whey protein powder, flaxseed meal, and sugar substitute in a blender.

- Blend 30 seconds or until smooth.

Makes one 16-ounce smoothie.

Exchanges/Food Choices: 2 starch, 1 fruit, 1 1/2 fat-free milk, 2 medium-fat protein
Per serving: Calories 460, Calories from Fat 80, Total Fat 9 g, Saturated Fat 3 g,
Trans Fat 0 g, Cholesterol 60 mg, Sodium 260 mg, Potassium 870 mg,
Total Carbohydrate 63 g, Dietary Fiber 2 g, Sugars 56 g, Protein 33 g, Phosphorus 345 mg

Shopping List:

1 bottle 100% pomegranate juice, unsweetened
1 carton light vanilla soymilk
1 carton low-fat vanilla yogurt

Staples:

vanilla whey protein powder
flaxseed meal
sugar substitute

Shop Smart

- Light vanilla soymilk with 100 calories, 3.5 g fat, 6.0 g protein, 11.0 g carbohydrates (8.0 g sugar), 95 mg sodium per cup

- Low-fat vanilla or fruit-flavored yogurt (not fruit on the bottom) with 208 calories, 3.1 g fat, 12.1 g protein, 33.8 g carbohydrates, 162 mg sodium per cup

- Vanilla whey protein powder with 80 calories, 1.1 g fat, 16.0 g protein, 1.0 g carbohydrates, 65 mg sodium per 3/4 ounce

- Flaxseed meal with 37 calories, 2.9 g fat, 1.3 g protein, 2.0 g carbohydrates per tablespoon

- Sugar substitute of your choice (I have used several different brands in creating the recipes.)

Popeye Smoothie

Banana and ginger add an intriguing flavor to this spinach-based smoothie. Popeye would be proud to drink it.

Helpful Hints

■ This smoothie is best made just before needed.

2 cups washed, ready-to-eat spinach
3/4 cup ripe banana, sliced
1 tablespoon peeled fresh ginger, cut into small pieces
1 scoop (3/4 ounce) vanilla whey protein powder
2 tablespoons nonfat sour cream
1/4 cup toasted wheat germ
1/2 cup pasteurized, liquid egg whites

■ Place spinach, banana, ginger, whey protein powder, sour cream, wheat germ, and egg whites in a blender.

■ Blend 45 seconds or until smooth.

Makes one 8-ounce smoothie.

Exchanges/Food Choices: 1 starch, 2 fruit, 1 vegetable, 5 lean protein
Per serving: Calories 410, Calories from Fat 50, Total Fat 5 g, Saturated Fat 1.5 g,
Trans Fat 0 g, Cholesterol 50 mg, Sodium 380 mg, Potassium 1080 mg,
Total Carbohydrate 54 g, Dietary Fiber 10 g, Sugars 18 g,
Protein 42 g, Phosphorus 400 mg

Shopping List:

1 small bag washed, ready-to-eat spinach
1 ripe banana
1 small piece fresh ginger
1 carton nonfat sour cream

Staples:

vanilla whey protein powder
toasted wheat germ
pasteurized, egg whites

Shop Smart

- Vanilla whey protein powder with 80 calories, 1.1 g fat, 16.0 g protein, 1.0 g carbohydrates, 65 mg sodium per 3/4 ounce
- Nonfat sour cream with 9 calories, 0.4 g protein, 1.9 g carbohydrates, 17 mg sodium per tablespoon
- Toasted wheat germ with 27 calories, 0.8 g fat, 2.0 g protein, 3.5 g carbohydrates, 0 mg sodium per tablespoon
- Pasteurized, liquid egg whites with 6 calories, 1.0 g fat, 1.0 g protein, 11 mg sodium per tablespoon

Pumpkin Pleaser Smoothie

*Pumpkin with sweet spices gives a hint of autumn
and the holiday season to this smoothie.*

Helpful Hints

- Be sure pumpkin purée is without added spices.

3/4 cup canned pumpkin
1 cup fat-free milk
1/4 teaspoon ground cinnamon
1/8 teaspoon ground nutmeg
1/8 teaspoon ground ginger
Sugar substitute equivalent to 2 teaspoons sugar
2 teaspoons honey
1 tablespoon unsalted pecans (1/4 ounce)
1 tablespoon reduced-fat mayonnaise
1 slice whole-wheat bread (1 ounce)
1 ounce low-salt sliced deli turkey breast

- Place pumpkin, milk, cinnamon, nutmeg, ginger, sugar substitute, honey, and pecans in a blender.

- Blend 45 seconds or until smooth.

- Spread mayonnaise on bread and top with turkey. Serve with smoothie.

Makes one 16-ounce smoothie.

*Exchanges/Food Choices: 3 1/2 starch, 1 fat-free milk, 1 lean protein
Per serving: Calories 380, Calories from Fat 100, Total Fat 11 g, Saturated Fat 2 g,
Trans Fat 0 g, Cholesterol 20 mg, Sodium 560 mg, Potassium 940 mg,
Total Carbohydrate 54 g, Dietary Fiber 8 g, Sugars 34 g, Protein 21 g, Phosphorus 440 mg*

Shopping List:

1 can pumpkin purée
1 container ground nutmeg
1 container ground ginger
1 package unsalted pecans (1/4 ounce)
1 ounce low-salt sliced deli turkey
   breast

Staples:

fat-free milk
ground cinnamon
sugar substitute
honey
reduced-fat mayonnaise
whole-wheat bread

Shop Smart

- Sugar substitute of your choice (I have used several different brands in creating the recipes.)

Red Pepper Popper Smoothie

Ripe tomato and red bell pepper create a rich, thick smoothie. Add an open-face turkey sandwich to complete this tasty lunch.

Helpful Hints

- Toasted wheat germ lends a slightly nutty flavor. Regular wheat germ can be used.
- One half tablespoon of tomato paste is needed. It freezes well. Place the remaining amount in a freezer container and freeze for another use.

1/2 cup tomato cubes
1/2 cup sliced red bell pepper
1/4 cup fat-free, low-sodium chicken broth
1/2 cup low-fat cottage cheese, no salt added
1 teaspoon olive oil
1/2 tablespoon tomato paste
1 tablespoon toasted wheat germ
Sugar substitute equivalent to 2 teaspoons sugar
1 tablespoon reduced-fat mayonnaise
1 slice whole-wheat bread (1 ounce)
1 ounce low-salt, lean deli turkey breast

- Add tomato cubes, red bell pepper slices, chicken broth, cottage cheese, olive oil, tomato paste, wheat germ, and sugar substitute to a blender.
- Blend 30 seconds or until smooth.
- Spread mayonnaise on the bread and top with turkey.

Makes one 8-ounce smoothie.

Exchanges/Food Choices: 2 starch, 2 vegetable, 3 lean protein, 1 fat
Per serving: Calories 340, Calories from Fat 100, Total Fat 11 g, Saturated Fat 2 g,
Trans Fat 0 g, Cholesterol 20 mg, Sodium 430 mg, Potassium 780 mg,
Total Carbohydrate 34 g, Dietary Fiber 7 g, Sugars 12 g, Protein 29 g, Phosphorus 410 mg

Shopping List:

1 tomato
1 red bell pepper
1 carton low-fat cottage cheese, no salt
   added
1 small can tomato paste
1 jar toasted wheat germ
1 ounce low-salt, lean deli turkey breast

Staples:

fat-free, low-sodium chicken broth
olive oil
sugar substitute
reduced-fat mayonnaise
whole-wheat bread

Shop Smart

- Low-fat, no-salt-added cottage cheese with 163 calories, 2.3 g fat, 28.0 g protein, 6.1 g carbohydrates, 29 mg sodium per cup
- Toasted wheat germ with 27 calories, 0.8 g fat, 2.0 g protein, 3.5 g carbohydrates, 0 mg sodium per tablespoon
- Sugar substitute of your choice (I have used several different brands in creating the recipes.)

Vanilla Smoothie

Simple, pure vanilla flavor makes this a quick and delicious smoothie.

Helpful Hints

- Ground flaxseed can be used instead of flaxseed meal.
- To add extra flavor open a vanilla bean pod and scrape some of the vanilla seeds onto the top of the smoothie once it is poured into a glass.
- Store flaxseed in the refrigerator to keep it from becoming rancid.

1 cup nonfat vanilla yogurt
1 teaspoon vanilla extract
1 scoop (3/4 ounce) vanilla whey protein powder
2 tablespoons flaxseed meal
1 cup light vanilla soymilk (such as Silk)
Sugar substitute equivalent to 2 teaspoons sugar
1 cup ice cubes

- Place yogurt, vanilla extract, whey protein powder, flaxseed, soymilk, and sugar substitute in a blender.
- Blend 20 seconds or until smooth.
- Add ice cubes and blend 30 seconds or until thick.

Makes one 16-ounce smoothie.

Exchanges/Food Choices: 1 fat-free milk, 2 1/2 carbohydrate, 3 lean protein
Per serving: Calories 340, Calories from Fat 90, Total Fat 10 g, Saturated Fat 1.5 g,
Trans Fat 0 g, Cholesterol 50 mg, Sodium 280 mg, Potassium 910 mg,
Total Carbohydrate 32 g, Dietary Fiber 5 g, Sugars 24 g, Protein 33 g, Phosphorus 535 mg

Shopping List:

1 carton nonfat vanilla yogurt
1 carton light vanilla soymilk

Staples:

vanilla extract
vanilla whey protein powder
flaxseed meal
sugar substitute

Shop Smart

- Vanilla whey protein powder with 80 calories, 1.1 g fat, 16.0 g protein, 1.0 g carbohydrates, 65 mg sodium per 3/4 ounce
- Nonfat vanilla or fruit-flavored yogurt with 140 calories, 16.0 g protein, 17.0 g carbohydrates, 75 mg sodium per 6-ounce carton
- Flaxseed meal with 37 calories, 2.9 g fat, 1.3 g protein, 2.0 g carbohydrates per tablespoon
- Light vanilla soymilk with 60 calories, 1.5 g fat, 6.0 g protein, 6.0 g carbohydrates (4.0 g sugar), 125 mg sodium per cup (such as Silk)
- Sugar substitute of your choice (I have used several different brands in creating the recipes.)

TomatOJ Smoothie

Adding orange juice to tomatoes gives them an intriguing, sweet taste.

Helpful Hints

- A quick way to chop scallions is to snip them with a scissors.
- This smoothie is best when served immediately.

> 1 cup fresh tomato cubes
> 1/2 cup orange juice
> 1/3 cup snipped scallions
> 1 cup nonfat ricotta cheese
> 2 teaspoons olive oil
> Sugar substitute equivalent to 2 teaspoons sugar

- Place tomatoes, orange juice, scallions, ricotta cheese, olive oil, and sugar substitute in a blender.

- Blend 45 seconds or until smooth.

Makes one 16-ounce smoothie.

Exchanges/Food Choices: 1 fruit, 1 fat-free milk, 2 vegetable, 3 lean protein
Per serving: Calories 340, Calories from Fat 90, Total Fat 10 g, Saturated Fat 1.5 g,
Trans Fat 0 g, Cholesterol 60 mg, Sodium 280 mg, Potassium 1370 mg,
Total Carbohydrate 35 g, Dietary Fiber 3 g, Sugars 28 g, Protein 27 g, Phosphorus 525 mg

Shopping List:

1 small ripe tomato
1 carton or bottle orange juice
1 bunch scallions
1 carton nonfat ricotta cheese

Staples:

olive oil
sugar substitute

Shop Smart

- Nonfat ricotta cheese with 200 calories, 20.0 g protein, 20.0 g carbohydrates, 260 mg sodium per cup
- Sugar substitute of your choice (I have used several different brands in creating the recipes.)

Snacks

Almond Coconut Smoothie

Banana, almonds, and coconut combine to make this light, flavorful smoothie.

Helpful Hints

■ Look for unsweetened almond milk. It can be found in health food markets.

3/4 cup ripe banana, sliced
1 cup light, unsweetened almond milk
1/4 teaspoon ground cinnamon
1 scoop (3/4 ounce) vanilla whey protein powder
1 tablespoon desiccated coconut flakes (sweetened)

■ Add banana, almond milk, cinnamon, whey protein powder, and coconut to a blender.

■ Blend 45 seconds or until smooth.

Makes one 16-ounce smoothie.

Exchanges/Food Choices: 2 fruit, 1 carbohydrate, 3 1/2 lean protein
Per serving: Calories 300, Calories from Fat 70, Total Fat 8 g, Saturated Fat 2.5 g,
Trans Fat 0 g, Cholesterol 50 mg, Sodium 80 mg, Potassium 840 mg,
Total Carbohydrate 35 g, Dietary Fiber 8 g, Sugars 17 g, Protein 27 g, Phosphorus 30 mg

Shopping List:

1 ripe banana
1 carton light, unsweetened almond milk
1 small package desiccated coconut
   flakes (sweetened)

Staples:

ground cinnamon
vanilla whey protein powder

Shop Smart

■ Unsweetened almond milk with 3.0 g fat and 2.0 g carbohydrates per cup
■ Vanilla whey protein powder with 80 calories, 1.1 g fat, 16.0 g protein, 1.0 g carbohydrates, 65 mg sodium per 3/4 ounce
■ Desiccated coconut flakes (sweetened) with 388 calories, 24.0 g fat, 44.1 g carbohydrates, 242 mg sodium per cup

Apple Pie Perfect

Apples and cinnamon create the aroma and flavors of an all-American apple pie. Sipping this smoothie brought back memories of stuffed apples baking in the oven on cool autumn days. Look for an apple-flavored, nonfat yogurt for this recipe.

Helpful Hints

- Precut apple slices are available in many supermarket produce sections. These work very well for this smoothie.
- Any variety of apple can be used.

> 1/3 cup apple slices
> 1/3 cup nonfat apple-flavored yogurt
> 1 tablespoon broken unsalted walnuts
> 1/2 teaspoon cinnamon
> Sugar substitute equivalent to 2 teaspoons sugar
> 1/4 cup water
> 1 cup ice cubes

- Place apple slices, yogurt, walnuts, cinnamon, sugar substitute, and water in a blender.

- Blend about 30 seconds.

- Add ice cubes.

- Blend about 30 seconds or until smooth.

Makes one 16-ounce smoothie.

Exchanges/Food Choices: 1 fruit, 1/2 fat-free milk, 2 fat
Per serving: Calories 190, Calories from Fat 90, Total Fat 10 g, Saturated Fat 1 g,
Trans Fat 0 g, Cholesterol <5 mg, Sodium 60 mg, Potassium 180 mg,
Total Carbohydrate 22 g, Dietary Fiber 3 g, Sugars 16 g, Protein 5 g, Phosphorus 100 mg

Shopping List:

1 small apple
1 small container nonfat apple-flavored
   yogurt
1 small package broken unsalted walnuts

Staples:

ground cinnamon
sugar substitute

Shop Smart

■ Nonfat vanilla or fruit-flavored yogurt with 140 calories, 16.0 g protein, 17.0 g carbohydrates, 75 mg sodium per 6-ounce carton

■ Sugar substitute of your choice (I have used several different brands in creating the recipes.)

Chai Spice 'n' Nice Smoothie (Green Tea Chai Smoothie)

Chai is a spiced-milk tea from India. Sweet spices mixed with green tea capture the flavors of this sweet drink for this smoothie.

Helpful Hints

- Hot water from an instant hot water faucet can be used instead of heating the water in a microwave oven.

1/2 teaspoon ground cinnamon
1/2 teaspoon ground ginger
1/2 cup water
1 green tea bag
3/4 cup light vanilla soymilk (such as Silk)
1 scoop (3/4 ounce) vanilla whey protein powder
Sugar substitute equivalent to 2 teaspoons sugar

- Place cinnamon, ginger, and water in a cup. Microwave on high 30 seconds. Remove cup from microwave and add tea bag.

- Steep tea 2 minutes.

- Place soymilk, whey protein powder, and sugar substitute in a blender. Remove tea bag and add tea to blender. Blend 30 seconds or until smooth.

Makes one 16-ounce smoothie.

Exchanges/Food Choices: 2 lean protein, 1 fat-free milk
Per serving: Calories 170, Calories from Fat 35, Total Fat 3.5 g, Saturated Fat 1 g,
Trans Fat 0 g, Cholesterol 50 mg, Sodium 120 mg, Potassium 180 mg,
Total Carbohydrate 12 g, Dietary Fiber 1 g, Sugars 8 g, Protein 21 g, Phosphorus 5 mg

Shopping List:

1 small container ground ginger
1 box green tea bags
1 small carton light vanilla soymilk

Staples:

ground cinnamon
vanilla whey protein powder
sugar substitute

Shop Smart

- Light vanilla soymilk with 70 calories, 1.5 g fat, 6.0 g protein, 7.0 g carbohydrates (5.0 g sugar), 110 mg sodium per cup (such as Silk)
- Vanilla whey protein powder with 80 calories, 1.1 g fat, 16.0 g protein, 1.0 g carbohydrates, 65 mg sodium per 3/4 ounce
- Sugar substitute of your choice (I have used several different brands in creating the recipes.)

Citrus Surprise Smoothie

Orange and grapefruit segments make this a sunny, mid-afternoon snack.

Helpful Hints

- If available, use low-fat orange yogurt instead of low-fat vanilla yogurt for an added orange flavor.
- For faster preparation, buy fresh, unsweetened orange and grapefruit segments in the produce section.

1/2 cup orange segments
1/2 cup grapefruit segments
1/2 cup low-fat vanilla yogurt
1/2 cup pasteurized, liquid egg whites
Sugar substitute equivalent to 2 teaspoons sugar
1/4 teaspoon orange extract
1/2 cup ice cubes

- Place orange segments, grapefruit segments, yogurt, egg whites, sugar substitute, and orange extract in a blender.

- Blend 30 seconds.

- Add the ice cubes and blend 30 seconds or until smooth.

Makes one 16-ounce smooth.

Exchanges/Food Choices: 1 fat-free milk, 2 carbohydrate, 2 lean protein
Per serving: Calories 170, Calories from Fat 25, Total Fat 3 g, Saturated Fat 1 g,
Trans Fat 0 g, Cholesterol 5 mg, Sodium 280 mg, Potassium 600 mg,
Total Carbohydrate 40 g, Dietary Fiber 3 g, Sugars 36 g, Protein 21 g, Phosphorus 190 mg

Shopping List:

1 orange or orange segments
1 grapefruit or grapefruit segments
1 carton low-fat vanilla yogurt
1 bottle orange extract

Staples:

pasteurized, liquid egg whites
sugar substitute

Shop Smart

■ Low-fat vanilla or fruit-flavored yogurt (not fruit on the bottom) with 208 calories, 3.1 g fat, 12.1 g protein, 33.8 g carbohydrates, 162 mg sodium per cup

■ Pasteurized, liquid egg whites with 6 calories, 1.0 g fat, 1.0 g protein, 11 mg sodium per tablespoon

■ Sugar substitute of your choice (I have used several different brands in creating the recipes.)

Coffee Coconut Smoothie

Coffee with a hint of coconut takes on the taste of the tropics.
It's a quick, pick-me-up drink. Serve immediately.

Helpful Hints

- Use powdered, instant regular or decaffeinated coffee. Do not mix it with water.
- Coconut extract can be found in the spice section of the supermarket.

2 teaspoons instant coffee
1/2 cup pasteurized, liquid egg whites
1/8 teaspoon coconut extract
Sugar substitute equivalent to 2 teaspoons sugar
1/2 cup water

- Place instant coffee, egg whites, coconut extract, sugar substitute, and water in a blender.
- Blend 30 seconds or until smooth.

Makes one 16-ounce smoothie.

Exchanges/Food Choices: 2 lean protein
Per serving: Calories 80, Calories from Fat 0, Total Fat 0 g, Saturated Fat 0 g,
Trans Fat 0 g, Cholesterol 0 mg, Sodium 210 mg, Potassium 130 mg,
Total Carbohydrate 4 g, Dietary Fiber <1 g, Sugars 0 g, Protein 14 g, Phosphorus 10 mg

Shopping List:

1 jar instant coffee
1 bottle coconut extract

Staples:

pasteurized, liquid egg whites
sugar substitute

Shop Smart

- Pasteurized, liquid egg whites with 6 calories, 1.0 g fat, 1.0 g protein, 11 mg sodium per tablespoon
- Sugar substitute of your choice (I have used several different brands in creating the recipes.)

Cranberry, Orange, and Banana Smoothie

Cranberries make this a tart and refreshing smoothie.
The bananas add a sweet finish.

Helpful Hints

■ Frozen or fresh cranberries work well in this smoothie.

> 1/4 cup fresh or frozen cranberries
> 1/4 cup ripe banana, sliced
> 1/4 cup orange juice
> 2 tablespoons pasteurized, liquid egg whites
> Sugar substitute equivalent to 2 teaspoons sugar
> 1/4 cup ice cubes

■ Place cranberries, banana, orange juice, egg whites, and sugar substitute in a blender. Blend 30 seconds.

■ Add the ice cubes. Blend 30 seconds or until smooth.

Makes one 8-ounce smoothie.

Exchanges/Food Choices: 1 fruit, 1/2 very lean protein
Per serving: Calories 90, Calories from Fat 0, Total Fat 0 g, Saturated Fat 0 g,
Trans Fat 0 g, Cholesterol 0 mg, Sodium 50 mg, Potassium 280 mg,
Total Carbohydrate 19 g, Dietary Fiber 2 g, Sugars 11 g, Protein 4 g, Phosphorus 20 mg

Shopping List:

1 package cranberries
1 ripe banana
1 container orange juice

Staples:

pasteurized, liquid egg whites
sugar substitute

Shop Smart

■ Pasteurized, liquid egg whites with 6 calories, 1.0 g fat, 1.0 g protein, 11 mg sodium per tablespoon

■ Sugar substitute of your choice (I have used several different brands in creating the recipes.)

Cucumber Melon Refresher Smoothie

The unusual combination of honeydew melon and cucumber blends together to make a crisp, sweet, refreshing smoothie.

Helpful Hints

- You can save a little preparation time by buying honeydew melon cubes that are ready to eat in the produce section of the supermarket.
- Firm tofu can be used instead of soft.
- To remove cucumber seeds, cut the cucumber in half lengthwise and then in quarters lengthwise. Slice off the seeds.

> 1 1/2 cups honeydew melon, cubed
> 1 cup cucumber, peeled, seeded, and cubed
> 1/2 cup soft tofu
> Sugar substitute equivalent to 2 teaspoons sugar

- Place melon, cucumber, tofu, and sugar substitute in a blender.
- Blend for 45 seconds or until smooth.

Makes one 12-ounce smoothie.

Exchanges/Food Choices: 2 fruit, 1 1/2 medium-fat protein
Per serving: Calories 180, Calories from Fat 45, Total Fat 5 g, Saturated Fat 1 g,
Trans Fat 0 g, Cholesterol 0 mg, Sodium 60 mg, Potassium 910 mg,
Total Carbohydrate 30 g, Dietary Fiber 3 g, Sugars 24 g, Protein 10 g, Phosphorus 170 mg

Shopping List:

1 ripe honeydew melon
1 cucumber
1 package soft tofu

Staples:

sugar substitute

Shop Smart

- Soft tofu with 151 calories, 9.2 g fat, 16.2 g protein, 4.5 g carbohydrates, 20 mg sodium per cup
- Sugar substitute of your choice (I have used several different brands in creating the recipes.)

Cucumber Mint Cooler

Cool and refreshing with a hint of mint, this smoothie is a refreshing, savory snack.

Helpful Hints

- An easy way to chop mint is to snip the leaves from the stem with a scissors.
- To remove cucumber seeds, cut the cucumber in half lengthwise and then in quarters lengthwise. Slice off the seeds.

1/4 cup water
1 cup cucumber, peeled, seeded, and cubed
1/2 cup low-fat plain yogurt
2 tablespoons pasteurized, liquid egg whites
2 tablespoons snipped fresh mint

- Place water, cucumber, yogurt, egg whites, and mint in a blender.

- Blend 30 seconds or until smooth.

Makes one 10-ounce smoothie.

Exchanges/Food Choices: 1 fat-free milk, 1 1/2 lean protein
Per serving: Calories 120, Calories from Fat 20, Total Fat 2 g, Saturated Fat 1 g,
Trans Fat 0 g, Cholesterol 10 mg, Sodium 170 mg, Potassium 460 mg,
Total Carbohydrate 12 g, Dietary Fiber 1 g, Sugars 10 g, Protein 12 g, Phosphorus 200 mg

Shopping List:

1 small cucumber
1 carton low-fat plain yogurt
1 small bunch fresh mint

Staples:

pasteurized, liquid egg whites

Shop Smart

- Low-fat yogurt with 154 calories, 3.8 g fat, 12.9 g protein, 17.3 g carbohydrates, 172 mg sodium per cup
- Pasteurized, liquid egg whites with 6 calories, 1.0 g fat, 1.0 g protein, 11 mg sodium per tablespoon

Double Chocolate Raspberry Treat Smoothie

Chocolate and raspberries blend perfectly together with a rich chocolate flavor enhanced by the raspberries.

Helpful Hints

■ Make sure the cocoa powder is thoroughly mixed into the yogurt.

1 tablespoon cocoa powder, unsweetened
3/4 cup low-fat vanilla yogurt
3/4 cup light chocolate-flavored soymilk (such as Silk)
1/2 cup frozen, unsweetened raspberries
Sugar substitute equivalent to 2 teaspoons sugar

■ Mix the cocoa powder into the yogurt until completely blended.

■ Add to a blender along with the soymilk, raspberries, and sugar substitute.

■ Blend 30 seconds or until smooth.

Makes one 8-ounce smoothie.

Exchanges/Food Choices: 1/2 fruit, 1 fat-free milk, 1 carbohydrate
Per serving: Calories 210, Calories from Fat 35, Total Fat 4 g, Saturated Fat 2 g,
Trans Fat 0 g, Cholesterol 10 mg, Sodium 210 mg, Potassium 80 mg,
Total Carbohydrate 31 g, Dietary Fiber 5 g, Sugars 22 g, Protein 14 g, Phosphorus 40 mg

Shopping List:

1 package unsweetened cocoa powder
1 carton low-fat vanilla yogurt
1 carton light chocolate-flavored soymilk
1 package frozen, unsweetened
   raspberries

Staples:

sugar substitute

Shop Smart

- Low-fat vanilla or fruit-flavored yogurt (not fruit on the bottom) with 208 calories, 3.1 g fat, 12.1 g protein, 33.8 g carbohydrates, 162 mg sodium per cup
- Light chocolate-flavored soymilk with 90 calories, 1.5 g fat, 3.0 g protein, 16.0 g carbohydrates (14.0 g sugar), 85 mg sodium per cup (such as Silk)
- Sugar substitute of your choice (I have used several different brands in creating the recipes.)

Espresso Crema Smoothie

This coffee-flavored smoothie is perfect for a mid-afternoon pick me up.

Helpful Hints

■ Use powdered, instant regular or decaffeinated coffee. Do not mix it with water. If you like a strong coffee flavor, add another teaspoon of instant espresso coffee.

> 2 teaspoons instant espresso coffee
> 1/2 cup low-fat coffee-flavored yogurt
> Sugar substitute equivalent to 2 teaspoons sugar
> 1/2 cup water
> 1/2 cup ice cubes

■ Place instant espresso coffee, yogurt, sugar substitute, and water in a blender. Blend 30 seconds.

■ Add ice cubes. Blend 30 seconds or until smooth.

Makes one 16-ounce smoothie.

Exchanges/Food Choices: 1 fat-free milk, 1/2 other carbohydrate
Per serving: Calories 120, Calories from Fat 15, Total Fat 2 g, Saturated Fat 1 g,
Trans Fat 0 g, Cholesterol 10 mg, Sodium 80 mg, Potassium 400 mg,
Total Carbohydrate 22 g, Dietary Fiber <1 g, Sugars 18 g, Protein 5 g, Phosphorus 155 mg

Shopping List:

1 small jar instant espresso coffee
1 carton low-fat coffee-flavored yogurt

Staples:

sugar substitute

Shop Smart

■ Low-fat vanilla or fruit-flavored yogurt (not fruit on the bottom) with 208 calories, 3.1 g fat, 12.1 g protein, 33.8 g carbohydrates, 162 mg sodium per cup

■ Sugar substitute of your choice (I have used several different brands in creating the recipes.)

Ginger-Limeade Smoothie

The combination of tangy lime juice, ginger ale, and creamy vanilla yogurt make a frothy, tangy smoothie.

Helpful Hints

- Any brand of diet ginger ale can be used. Look for 0 carbohydrates on the nutritional label.
- Remove the zest from the lime before cutting open to juice it.

1/2 tablespoon lime zest (grated skin)
2 tablespoons fresh lime juice
3/4 cup diet ginger ale
1 cup low-fat vanilla yogurt
Sugar substitute equivalent to 2 teaspoons sugar

- Add the lime zest, lime juice, ginger ale, yogurt, and sugar substitute to a blender.
- Blend 45 seconds or until smooth.

Makes one 16-ounce smoothie.

Exchanges/Food Choices: 1 fat-free milk, 1 1/2 carbohydrate
Per serving: Calories 210, Calories from Fat 30, Total Fat 3 g, Saturated Fat 2 g,
Trans Fat 0 g, Cholesterol 10 mg, Sodium 220 mg, Potassium 570 mg,
Total Carbohydrate 36 g, Dietary Fiber 0 g, Sugars 34 g, Protein 12 g, Phosphorus 335 mg

Shopping List:

1 lime
1 small bottle or can diet ginger ale
1 carton low-fat vanilla yogurt

Staples:

sugar substitute

Shop Smart

- Low-fat vanilla or fruit-flavored yogurt (not fruit on the bottom) with 208 calories, 3.1 g fat, 12.1 g protein, 33.8 g carbohydrates, 162 mg sodium per cup
- Sugar substitute of your choice (I have used several different brands in creating the recipes.)

Grape Escape Smoothie

Grapes enhanced with a little grape spread make a tasty, deep-purple smoothie.

Helpful Hints

- Look for low-sugar grape spread in the jam and jelly section of the market (8.0 g sugar per tablespoon).

> 1/4 cup water
> 1/2 cup low-fat vanilla yogurt
> 1/2 cup seedless red grapes
> 1 tablespoon low-sugar grape spreadable fruit (such as Welch's)
> 1 scoop (3/4 ounce) vanilla whey protein powder

- Place water, yogurt, grapes, grape spread, and whey protein powder in a blender.

- Blend 45 seconds or until smooth.

Makes one 12-ounce smoothie.

Exchanges/Food Choices: 1 fruit, 1 fat-free milk, 1 carbohydrate, 2 lean protein
Per serving: Calories 270, Calories from Fat 30, Total Fat 3 g, Saturated Fat 2 g,
Trans Fat 0 g, Cholesterol 55 mg, Sodium 120 mg, Potassium 530 mg,
Total Carbohydrate 38 g, Dietary Fiber 1 g, Sugars 34 g, Protein 223 g, Phosphorus 180 mg

Shopping List:

1 carton low-fat vanilla yogurt
1 small bunch seedless red grapes
1 jar low-sugar grape spreadable fruit
   (such as Welch's)

Staples:

vanilla whey protein powder

Shop Smart

- Low-fat vanilla or fruit-flavored yogurt (not fruit on the bottom) with 208 calories, 3.1 g fat, 12.1 g protein, 33.8 g carbohydrates, 162 mg sodium per cup
- Spreadable fruit with 30 calories, 8.0 g carbohydrates per tablespoon
- Vanilla whey protein powder with 80 calories, 1.1 g fat, 16.0 g protein, 1.0 g carbohydrates, 65 mg sodium per 3/4 ounce

Guacamole Shake

Creamy, ripe avocado mixed with green pepper and hot sauce makes this a spicy, smoothie snack.

Helpful Hints

- The easiest way to chop chives is to snip them with a scissors.
- Make sure the avocado is ripe. It should give slightly when pressed with your thumb.

1/2 cup ripe California (Hass-type) avocado, cubed
1/2 cup green bell pepper, diced
1/4 cup fat-free milk
3 tablespoons pasteurized, liquid egg whites
2 tablespoons snipped chives
Several drops hot pepper sauce
Salt and freshly ground black pepper to taste

- Place avocado, green pepper, milk, egg whites, chives, and hot sauce in a blender.

- Blend 45 seconds or until smooth.

- Add salt and pepper to taste.

Makes one 8-ounce smoothie.

Exchanges/Food Choices: 1 carbohydrate, 1 lean protein, 1 fat
Per serving: Calories 180, Calories from Fat 100, Total Fat 10 g, Saturated Fat 2 g,
Trans Fat 0 g, Cholesterol <5 mg, Sodium 310 mg, Potassium 600 mg,
Total Carbohydrate 14 g, Dietary Fiber 6 g, Sugars 5 g, Protein 9 g, Phosphorus 120 mg

Shopping List:

1 small, ripe California (Hass-type) avocado
1 green bell pepper
1 bunch chives
1 small bottle hot pepper sauce

Staples:

fat-free milk
pasteurized, liquid egg whites
salt and black peppercorns

Shop Smart

- Pasteurized, liquid egg whites with 6 calories, 1.0 g fat, 1.0 g protein, 11 mg sodium per tablespoon

Lemon Cheesecake Shake

This smoothie is sweet, tart, lemony, and creamy.

Helpful Hints

- For added lemon zing, grate some lemon zest (grated lemon rind) on top of the smoothie just before serving.

1 tablespoon lemon zest (grated lemon rind)
2 tablespoons fresh lemon juice
1/4 teaspoon lemon extract
1/2 cup nonfat ricotta cheese
1/2 cup water
Sugar substitute equivalent to 3 teaspoons sugar
1/2 teaspoon ground cinnamon
1 tablespoon unsalted pecan pieces
1/2 cup ice cubes

- Place lemon zest, lemon juice, lemon extract, ricotta cheese, water, sugar substitute, ground cinnamon, and pecans in a blender.

- Blend 45 seconds.

- Add ice cubes.

- Blend 30 seconds or until smooth.

Makes one 8-ounce smoothie.

Exchanges/Food Choices: 1 low-fat milk, 1 lean protein, 1 fat
Per serving: Calories 140, Calories from Fat 45, Total Fat 5 g, Saturated Fat 0 g,
Trans Fat 0 g, Cholesterol 30 mg, Sodium 300 mg, Potassium 380 mg,
Total Carbohydrate 12 g, Dietary Fiber 2 g, Sugars 7 g, Protein 13 g, Phosphorus 250 mg

Shopping List:

2 lemons
1 small bottle lemon extract
1 small container nonfat ricotta cheese
1 small package unsalted pecans pieces

Staples:

sugar substitute
ground cinnamon

Shop Smart

- Nonfat ricotta cheese with 200 calories, 20.0 g protein, 20.0 g carbohydrates, 260 mg sodium per cup
- Sugar substitute of your choice (I have used several different brands in creating the recipes.)

Key Lime Smoothie

Key lime juice and yogurt create the flavors of the Florida Keys for this smoothie.

Helpful Hints

- Bottled key lime juice can be found in most supermarkets. Be sure to look for key lime juice not marinade.
- Fresh lime juice can be used if key lime juice is not available.

> 1/2 cup low-fat vanilla yogurt
> 2 tablespoons bottled key lime juice
> Sugar substitute equivalent to 2 teaspoons sugar
> 3/4 cup water
> 1/2 cup ice cubes

- Place yogurt, lime juice, sugar substitute, and water in a blender.
- Blend 30 seconds.
- Add ice cubes.
- Blend 30 seconds or until smooth.

Makes one 16-ounce smoothie.

Exchanges/Food Choices: 1 fat-free milk, 1/2 carbohydrate
Per serving: Calories 110, Calories from Fat 15, Total Fat 1.5 g, Saturated Fat 1 g,
Trans Fat 0 g, Cholesterol 5 mg, Sodium 90 mg, Potassium 300 mg,
Total Carbohydrate 21 g, Dietary Fiber 0 g, Sugars 17 g, Protein 6 g, Phosphorus 170 mg

Shopping List: ## Staples:

1 small carton low-fat vanilla yogurt   sugar substitute
1 small bottle key lime juice

Shop Smart

- Low-fat vanilla or fruit-flavored yogurt (not fruit on the bottom) with 208 calories, 3.1 g fat, 12.1 g protein, 33.8 g carbohydrates, 162 mg sodium per cup
- Sugar substitute of your choice (I have used several different brands in creating the recipes.)

Lemonade Lift Smoothie

This smoothie is as fresh as a summer breeze and light and tart.

Helpful Hints

- Look for frozen lemonade concentrate in the freezer section of the supermarket.

> 1 cup nonfat vanilla yogurt
> 3 tablespoons lemon juice
> 1 tablespoon (1/2 ounce) frozen lemonade concentrate
> 3/4 cup water
> 2 tablespoons dry-roasted cashew nuts with no added salt
> Sugar substitute equivalent to 3 teaspoons sugar

- Place yogurt, lemon juice, lemonade concentrate, water, cashew nuts, and sugar substitute in a blender.

- Blend 40–45 seconds or until smooth.

Makes one 16-ounce smoothie.

Exchanges/Food Choices: 1 1/2 fruit, 1 1/2 fat-free milk, 1 1/2 fat
Per serving: Calories 270, Calories from Fat 70, Total Fat 8 g, Saturated Fat 1.5 g,
Trans Fat 0 g, Cholesterol 0 mg, Sodium 160 mg, Potassium 150 mg,
Total Carbohydrate 40 g, Dietary Fiber 1 g, Sugars 34 g, Protein 13 g, Phosphorus 90 mg

Shopping List:

1 container nonfat vanilla yogurt
2 lemons
1 container frozen lemonade concentrate
1 package dry-roasted cashew nuts
   without added salt

Staples:

sugar substitute

Shop Smart

- Lemonade frozen concentrate with 72 calories, 18.2 g carbohydrates per fluid ounce
- Nonfat yogurt with 103 calories, 4.0 g fat, 9.3 g protein, 18.1 g carbohydrates, 142 mg sodium per cup
- Sugar substitute of your choice (I have used several different brands in creating the recipes.)

Orange Froth Smoothie

This is a light and frothy orange drink.

Helpful Hints

- For faster preparation, buy orange segments in the supermarket.
- An easy way to segment oranges is to cut into the skin just down to the flesh from the tip of the orange to the bottom. Make a second cut about 2 inches from the first. Peel the skin away and cut out the segment.

1/4 cup orange segments
1/2 cup diet orange soda
2 tablespoons pasteurized, liquid egg whites
Sugar substitute equivalent to 2 teaspoons sugar

- Place orange segments, orange soda, egg whites, and sugar substitute in a blender.
- Blend for 45 seconds or until smooth.

Makes one 10-ounce smoothie.

Exchanges/Food Choices: 1/2 fruit, 1/2 lean protein
Per serving: Calories 45, Calories from Fat 0, Total Fat 0 g, Saturated Fat 0 g,
Trans Fat 0 g, Cholesterol 0 mg, Sodium 75 mg, Potassium 130 mg,
Total Carbohydrate 8 g, Dietary Fiber 1 g, Sugars 6 g, Protein 4 g, Phosphorus 10 mg

Shopping List:

1 orange
1 small bottle or can diet orange soda

Staples:

pasteurized, liquid egg whites
sugar substitute

Shop Smart

- Diet soda with 0 calories and a range of 0–80 mg sodium per cup
- Pasteurized, liquid egg whites with 6 calories, 1.0 g fat, 1.0 g protein, 11 mg sodium per tablespoon
- Sugar substitute of your choice (I have used several different brands in creating the recipes.)

Peach Freeze Smoothie

This smoothie reminds me of summertime when the farmer's market stalls are filled with the unmistakable aroma of ripe peaches. Using frozen, unsweetened peach slices, you can enjoy this summer boost year round.

Helpful Hints

- Low-fat vanilla yogurt can be used if peach yogurt is not available.
- Firm tofu can be used instead of soft.

1/4 cup water
1/2 cup soft tofu
1 cup frozen, unsweetened peach slices
1/2 cup low-fat peach yogurt

- Place water, tofu, peach slices, and yogurt in a blender.

- Blend 45 seconds or until smooth.

Makes one 12-ounce smoothie.

Exchanges/Food Choices: 1 1/2 fruit, 1 fat-free milk, 1 medium-fat protein
Per serving: Calories 230, Calories from Fat 50, Total Fat 6 g, Saturated Fat 1.5 g,
Trans Fat 0 g, Cholesterol <5 mg, Sodium 90 mg, Potassium 150 mg,
Total Carbohydrate 37 g, Dietary Fiber 2 g, Sugars 31 g, Protein 13 g, Phosphorus 115 mg

Shopping List:

1 package soft tofu
1 package frozen, unsweetened peach
   slices
1 carton low-fat peach yogurt

Shop Smart

- Soft tofu with 151 calories, 9.2 g fat, 16.2 g protein, 4.5 g carbohydrates, 20 mg sodium per cup
- Low-fat vanilla or fruit-flavored yogurt (not fruit on the bottom) with 208 calories, 3.1 g fat, 12.1 g protein, 33.8 g carbohydrates, 162 mg sodium per cup

Virgin Piña Colada Smoothie

This smoothie has the flavors of a tropical piña colada without the added fat.

Helpful Hints

- Pineapple cubes are available in the produce department of the supermarket.

1/4 cup fresh pineapple cubes
1/4 cup light coconut milk
Sugar substitute equivalent to 2 teaspoons sugar
1 scoop (3/4 ounce) vanilla whey protein powder
1/8 teaspoon coconut extract
1/4 cup water
1/2 cup ice cubes

- Place pineapple cubes, coconut milk, sugar substitute, whey protein powder, coconut extract, and water in a blender. Blend 30 seconds.

- Add ice. Blend 30 seconds or until smooth.

Makes one 10-ounce smoothie.

Exchanges/Food Choices: 1 fruit, 2 lean protein, 1 fat
Per serving: Calories 130, Calories from Fat 20, Total Fat 3 g, Saturated Fat 2 g,
Trans Fat 0 g, Cholesterol 50 mg, Sodium 50 mg, Potassium 210 mg,
Total Carbohydrate 11 g, Dietary Fiber <1 g, Sugars 7 g, Protein 17 g, Phosphorus 25 mg

Shopping List:

1 small container fresh pineapple cubes
1 can light coconut milk
1 bottle coconut extract

Staples:

sugar substitute
vanilla whey protein powder

Shop Smart

- Light coconut milk with 135 calories, 13.3 g fat, 3.0 g protein, 9.0 g carbohydrates, 60.0 mg sodium per cup

- Vanilla whey protein powder with 80 calories, 1.1 g fat, 16.0 g protein, 1.0 g carbohydrates, 65 mg sodium per 3/4 ounce

- Sugar substitute of your choice (I have used several different brands in creating the recipes.)

Raspberry Banana Cooler

Sweet bananas, raspberries, almonds, and lemon-lime soda make this a fizzy treat.

Helpful Hints

■ Look for a diet lemon-lime soda without caffeine (such as diet Sprite).

> 1 cup frozen, unsweetened raspberries
> 1/2 cup ripe banana, sliced
> 1 cup diet lemon-lime soda
> 2 tablespoons sliced almonds
> Sugar substitute equivalent to 2 teaspoons sugar

■ Place raspberries, banana, soda, almonds, and sugar substitute in a blender.

■ Blend 45 seconds or until smooth.

Makes one 10-ounce smoothie.

Exchanges/Food Choices: 2 fruit, 1 fat
Per serving: Calories 180, Calories from Fat 50, Total Fat 6 g, Saturated Fat 0.5 g,
Trans Fat 0 g, Cholesterol 0 mg, Sodium 30 mg, Potassium 350 mg,
Total Carbohydrate 34 g, Dietary Fiber 8 g, Sugars 14 g, Protein 4 g, Phosphorus 70 mg

Shopping List:

1 package frozen, unsweetened
   raspberries
1 ripe banana
1 bottle or can diet lemon-lime soda
1 small package sliced almonds

Staples:

sugar substitute

Shop Smart

■ Diet soda with 0 calories and a range of 0–80 mg sodium per cup

■ Sugar substitute of your choice (I have used several different brands in creating the recipes.)

Index

G

I

K

L

M

N

O

P

T

V

W